*'Take me back to where the sky and sea collide,
where I knew in that moment we were infinite'*

Prologue

'Ssh!'

'What?'

'I think I can hear something.'

'You're imagining it.'

'I said, "Shh." I can't hear over you two talking.'

I cocked my ear towards the door. There was sometimes a telltale sign – the squeak of the living-room door hinge, the creak of the bottom stair, a squelch of a leather boot that might give some indication that *she* was approaching. If we all heard it at the same time we'd each be under the duvet without anyone having to sound the warning. It offered little to no protection, of course, but nevertheless we'd try to cover the most vulnerable parts of our bodies, the areas she always went for – the hair, stomach, legs. If one of us clocked something there might only be time to sound the alarm and duck for cover, leaving the others to fend for themselves. Not being quick enough to get under the

1

duvet could be fatal. As would being caught sitting up or, worse, out of bed. Even being caught before you could feign sleep, just lying there with one eye open, meant punishment. Who was I kidding? Like she needed an excuse. When someone metes out beatings for fun they'll come up with any reason to satisfy their lust.

We'd been silent for nearly a minute. Still nothing.

Just because I hadn't heard another sound meant little. She could still be waiting right outside the door, ready to pounce. She'd been known to wait several minutes just to catch us out. Tonight was a tricky one, though. She had guests in – her older children – who didn't know anything of what went on upstairs, just like Terry, her ever-trusting hubby. They'd never believe what she got up to. Not that sweet old lady. The one who wanted us to call her Granny. She wasn't capable of anything like that. They'd be like everyone else who didn't believe us. 'Nasty girls,' they'd think. 'Say anything for a bit of attention, they will. After all we do for the little wretches.'

But just because she was entertaining didn't mean she'd take her eye off the ball. There were no nights off. No respite. No easy rides in the Bad Room.

'Well?' Sara said. She always found it hardest to keep quiet. That was my fault. I'd brought her out of her shell a little. Before I was condemned to the Bad Room she was a little church mouse. She wasn't much older than me but you'd never tell from looking at us. Such a skinny thing, like her big sister, Arlene. Now *she* was a funny one; given how old she was – two years older than Sara – and that she towered over everyone in his house, including her sister, you'd think she might put up more of a fight. But she was like the dogs you saw on those animal cruelty adverts on TV, the ones with the haunted eyes that gave a glimpse of the terror they'd faced.

'Maybe nothing,' I said. I'd been in this place so long my mind played tricks on me.

'As I was saying,' Sara went on from where she was sitting on the top bunk above me, her bare legs swinging down, atop a duvet that was half pulled back for ease of entry. 'If this goes on we'll have to steal food from school tomorrow.'

'Me steal, more like,' I said, recalling the last time I'd swiped some muffins when we'd gone without food for a day. The mention of food brought on a pang of nausea, the memories of sweet choc-chip muffins made my mouth water. Today hadn't been too bad; we'd actually had breakfast. Nothing for lunch and she had played her game with dinner again; leaving a ham sandwich – if you could call it that – at the bottom of the stairs but neglecting to call us to get it, then making a big deal of punishing us for being ungrateful. 'If you lot don't want your dinner, that suits me fine. You can starve.'

Boy, did we starve. I couldn't tell you how much my stomach had shrunk since I'd moved here but it still hurt to go without. Gulping mouthfuls of water from the bathroom tap wasn't the same. Even if the sandwich was one sliver of wafer-thin ham on two tea biscuits it was like a royal banquet to us.

'I could steal too, you know.' Sara's soft voice came from above. I could picture her indignant frown. The legs stopped swinging.

'Yeah, right. You'd brick yourself.' I liked taking the mick out of her but the truth was I didn't want her to get into trouble. If I got caught it would only be me getting the flak. Like last time. I wouldn't want Sara to go through what I did when I got home and she had been waiting for me.

'Bloody could you know,' Sara had raised her voice above the acceptable level. I caught Arlene's eye. She knew we were taking a big risk talking this loudly. Sara carried on regardless: 'I'd bring back food for all …'

CRASH!

The door swung open so violently I thought it would break off its hinges.

Oh hell!

'Who's talking?!'

For a small lady she sure filled the doorway. I only caught a glimpse of black – the knee-high boots and that hair – before I dived undercover.

'You!'

Even under the duvet, my eyes were tight shut. I heard the scream over the smack on flesh. Sara. She'd never have made it under in time. Another scream, the shaking of the bunk beds, a yelp and a bang and scream combined. I didn't need to be watching to tell the nature of the violence. I knew well enough by the reaction. A slap to the thigh, a fistful of hair and a wrench that would have hauled Sara off her bunk down onto the floor. Definitely a sore one.

'I'll ask again. Who was talking?'

Don't say a word, Sara. Don't say a word. There was strength in numbers. We had to stick together. Pitting us against each other was the way she wanted it. I could hear whimpering. I imagined Sara's lip quivering. Another slap. The yell.

'You!' The sound of another smack on cotton. Most likely Arlene this time. Maybe a boot to her stomach or back, depending on how she was lying.

'So it's like that, is it?'

I pulled the duvet a little tighter around my head. My whole body was rigid. Sara was still whimpering, probably on the floor where she fell.

'I've told you to be quiet. Do you think I was born yesterday?'

Apart from the whimpering there was silence. *Good girl, Sara.*

'This isn't over.'

A shuffle towards the door, a pause, and then the door quietly closed shut.

It was done, for now. By her standards that was light. Perhaps it was a warning – just because she had family round we shouldn't think she wasn't still monitoring us.

I peeked out in time to see Sara, her face stained with tears, climbing unsteadily back to the top bunk.

'You okay?' I whispered.

She nodded. She'd done well. Months ago she would have blabbed, dobbed me in, even if it wasn't me doing the talking. But we'd turned a corner. They were all right really, these two. Not like it had been when I first came to the house. Back then I thought them weird. Sitting on the floor in their room with their night-dresses on, even though it was four o'clock in the after-noon. What was that all about? Not saying a word, at opposite ends of the room, either playing with a little bit of Lego or drawing shapes in a notepad. Other times when I went in – quickly, mind you, just to get some clothes out of the wardrobe – they'd be in bed. No wonder they were so pasty white.

'Thank God I'm not in there,' I'd thought at the time.

Back then, in 2001, I was only ten. I didn't know many things. But I knew you did not want to go in that room. You did not want to be a child in that room.

It was a Bad Room.

Then, without warning, I was in it too.

And I realised that I didn't have a clue. Life inside the Bad Room was way worse than even I had imagined. I needed to draw on all my strength just to get through every spirit-sapping day. I had to use all my wiles to survive.

Luckily, I had years of practice in that matter.

Violence, persecution and neglect were pretty much all I knew.

Chapter 1

Most children, I imagine, when they look back on their early childhood might remember a birthday party, a special Christmas or a fun-filled family holiday. Thinking back might conjure memories of Mum's warm cuddles, playing games with Dad and getting up to mischief with siblings.

I have tried to avoid delving too deeply into my childhood, because when I do it's not the fun times I focus on, as these were few and far between. Mostly I remember the violence, the neglect and the times spent living in fear. Then there are the feelings of wanting to be as far away as possible from my mum.

I was born in 1988 to Mandy Gallagher and James Matthews, two teenage sweethearts from a town in Greater Manchester who were far too young to be parents. Mum was only 17 and Dad just two years older. I have only the faintest recollections of them being together, as they split when I was 18 months old. It was like there was a brief moment when he was there and we were all together, then he wasn't and I had to go to a different house to see him.

If it was tough enough for two teenagers to adjust to being parents so young, they had the added torment of having to deal with the loss of a baby. That's because I was a twin. My sibling didn't make it. Mum didn't know she was expecting more than one. When she suffered a miscarriage, they were devastated. They hadn't detected me at the time. It was only when she went into hospital to get checked out that they told her, 'There's another one here.'

They had found a new heartbeat – mine.

For any young woman it would have been quite an ordeal, but she was still a child herself and had to deal with that loss and the turmoil of emotions it caused her. What made it doubly difficult for Mum was that there was no support from her own parents.

Mum had never known her own father. Her mother was originally from Ireland and when she fell pregnant it might as well have been to a man with no name. Mum had two brothers and a sister and their father was never spoken about. What made things even worse was that she endured a toxic relationship with her mum, my grandma.

Mum doted on her mum, craved her love and approval. Every piece of jewellery that my grandma had was from my mum. She spoiled her. Over the years she gave her new pieces each birthday, Mother's Day and Christmas, kitted out her whole house with stuff, but still my grandma seemed to favour the other children over her. Nothing she ever did was good enough. I know this, because she told me constantly, like she told me about my tragic twin. Mum had a habit of sharing this type of detail. She almost forgot that I was the child and spoke to me as an adult; she didn't treat me like a normal mum should. Sometimes I felt she didn't love me or that she wished my twin had survived. After all, she wasn't even aware I existed until she went to the hospital with complications. She'd had to overcome feelings of despair and then had to deal with being told there was another heartbeat. Perhaps she didn't bond with me properly, felt disconnected, and that affected our whole future relationship? We had conversations about stuff and I heard things that a child should never have heard. For instance, she told me that one time when she and her mother were arguing, Grandma held a razorblade to my mum's eyes. After that, Mum couldn't stand anything being held near her face.

Despite their volatile relationship, Grandma lived nearby and was always at our house. Four or five times a week we saw her. It was constant.

In contrast, my dad's side of the family was fantastic. He was a painter-decorator and worked hard. My grandad was called Richard and he ran a few convenience stores. In the early years after Mum and Dad split, Dad would pick me up every week and take me to one of the shops. I helped Grandad by putting the sweets out on the shelves, or he let me go behind the till and play shops for real. He had broken up with Dad's real mum when he was young as well and he lived with his wife, Heather. I never knew her as Grandma because Dad took me to visit his mum as well. She was my other Grandma. Dad had met a new woman shortly after splitting from my mum and they would take me out and make a fuss of me. They were a nice family.

My mum had two older brothers, William and Andrew. William lived locally and we saw a fair bit of him, but Andrew had left home at a young age and wasn't in our lives. Mum's younger sister was my Auntie Marie. She was the fun one, always hanging around our house and wanting to have a laugh. She couldn't have been prouder to be an auntie and always wanted to take me out in the pram or pushchair to show her friends. She was full of mischief. If Marie took me out on the bus she'd lead me to the back seat, and as Mum waved us off Marie would say things like, 'Stick your finger up at her.'

When we got home Mum would be furious and tell her off, but Marie just laughed. She once turned up with thirteen kittens she'd rescued from somewhere. They were so cute. I wanted to keep them all. Mum went ballistic, though, and said there was no way we were keeping all those cats. We had to give them all away.

At night sometimes, after she'd played with me all day, Marie climbed into bed with me. I loved it when she was around.

There were some nice qualities that Mum shared with her sister. Mum was house-proud and I remember our home was filled with photos, some professionally taken. She was a talented artist, too, and she sketched famous faces with ease. When it was my birthday she threw a party in McDonald's and there were other times when she liked to surprise me in the morning by laying a Kinder chocolate egg with the toys inside next to my bed. I was into the little porcelain green frogs that were popular at the time and I remember collecting them for my grandma's kitchen worktop.

So, even though Mum and Dad were not together, it wasn't all bad.

The trouble was, Mum never got over my dad leaving her, so there was always an atmosphere between them. I was a daddy's girl when I was little and I loved it when he came to pick me up. He had a lovely house and even at a young age I felt he had a better set-up than Mum. And when I went to Dad's I was always playing, going shopping, getting treats. That's often just how it is when two parents split up. Sometimes I couldn't help myself and would come home from a visit announcing that I wanted to go and live with him.

Mum was, perhaps understandably, bitter and jealous. Whenever I came back she interrogated me. 'What is his new woman like, what's the house like, what did they say about me?'

She was always very anxious, there was always an issue, always something she was kicking off about. That created a negative atmosphere and for as long as I can remember I could sense it was toxic.

Home for Mum and I was, for the most part, a first-floor council flat in an estate that's been much maligned in the media since it was built in the seventies. It's been called a 'welfare ghetto' because of the higher-than-average number of people living there on benefits.

Mum might have been one of the people trying to get by on benefits but to us it was home for a number of years. Our entire world was close at hand. Grandma lived on the next street; she ran a pub up the road, where Mum sometimes helped out. My Auntie Marie wasn't far away.

After my dad left, that was our set-up. I lived with Mum and got to see him at weekends. If the situation had remained like that maybe things would have been all right. But things rarely do stay the same.

Aside from these early details, I can't really remember any other significant good times with my mum. I don't know if I've blocked them out. I have memories of her being in a good mood, when there would be new clothes and presents, but I can't remember a load of affection.

Much of this was because by the time I was three Mum got involved with a new boyfriend. Paul Harries was 6ft 4in tall with a thick, dark moustache. From the moment he appeared on the scene he had an intimidating presence. Everyone wanted to please him because they were scared of him. They wanted to stay on his good side.

Everyone, except my mum, could see he was toxic. He was possessive and controlling but she worshipped the ground he walked on. What I didn't know at the time was that he was one of the town's biggest drug dealers.

I knew enough to know he was trouble, though. They might have loved each other, but when Mum and Paul kicked off it was chaos. And they kicked off a lot.

That's when the trouble started with my mum. Mentally, she began to fall apart.

And when the trouble started, I was caught in the middle of it all.

Chapter 2

'Come on,' Paul said, when he was looking after me one day, 'we're going to a friend's house.'

When we got there he left me to play with the other children while he and the two adults huddled in the kitchen around the cooker. I could see spoons, tin foil and little bags of sand. I might only have been four, and just a little child, but I observed everything and absorbed what was happening. I spent nearly all of my time around adults and I knew enough about their behaviour, the noises they made and the way they spoke to know when they were doing something wrong. Mum openly spoke about drugs and how much she was against Paul taking them. I saw one of the men hand Paul a bag of the sand. Was that the drugs she had been going on about?

We were in the house for quite a while. All the time I was playing with the other kids I kept an eye on Paul to see what he was up to. On the way home we stopped off at a shop and he bought me a teddy bear and an ice-lolly.

'If your mum asks us where we went, just say we went to my friend's and then to the park, okay?' he said, patting me on the head.

I nodded.

Later on when I was alone with my mum she sat me down and started firing questions at me.

'Where were you today? What did you get up to?'

I did what Paul said and told her we went to the park, but it was like she didn't believe me. She kept quizzing me over and over. Remembering what Paul said, I stayed quiet. Then she went in a mood with me. I hated it when she did that as all I wanted was for her to pay me attention and like me. The longer I kept quiet the angrier she became until she started yelling at me. I didn't think I had a choice so I told her what I'd seen at the house.

'Paul got some tiny bags of sand and I was not allowed to tell you.'

'Is that right?'

That night when Paul came home they had an almighty row. In my room I could hear them screaming at each other and the sounds of objects being thrown. When they had one of their arguments you did not want to be in the firing line. In the morning not a lot was being said between them. Paul got me ready to walk to the shops. On the way he held my hand.

'Why did you tell your mum what we got up to yesterday when I told you not to?' He spoke quietly but menacingly. He had my hand clasped between his thick fingers.

'Mum kept asking what we'd done. She didn't believe me.'

Paul began squeezing my fingers.

'The next time I tell you not to do something you'd better not do it.'

I tried to pull my hand away but he was gripping it too firmly. It tightened even more.

'Ow, you're hurting me!'

My hand felt like it was being crushed. I started to cry and finally he released his grip. We carried on to the shops in silence, apart from my sniffs and sobs, and all the time I was terrified he would do something else to hurt me. From that day on crushing my hand became a regular punishment; as well as slaps to my legs that stung so hot even thinking about it today brings back the burning sensation. Often he'd hit me so hard an imprint of his hand would remain on my leg. The slaps came without warning and I lived in a state of fear that at any moment he might erupt and another one would be heading my way.

Mum then told me that Paul took and sold drugs. She explained that the sand I had seen was actually heroin and the spoons and foil were used to cook the drugs before they took them. It wasn't the type of conversation a mum should be having with a four-year-old child, but she had no filter. At the time I didn't fully understand what she was saying but I knew it was something I wasn't to discuss with anyone else. At least Mum, to her credit, was very anti-drugs and most of their arguments were about whether he was still using.

I had always had the impression that Paul didn't like me because I was James's daughter, but after that incident he had a reason to dislike me even more. Even though he was cruel to me and he and Mum were constantly rowing, if anything, when he wasn't around life was worse. Often he would leave, go AWOL, or Mum would throw him out. But then, whenever that happened, Mum missed him and cried a lot. It felt like she was angry all the time and took her fury out on me. She'd hit me for no reason, scream at me over the tiniest thing and I'd never know what would set her off next time.

It got so unbearable that I often begged Mum to take him back because the beatings and the shouting at me were horrible. Paul was always persistent and he would show up claiming to have cleaned up his act and promising to be better. Mum, because she loved him, took him back every time.

Whenever Paul moved back in life would be calm for a little while. We'd sit and watch television together like a normal family, have Sunday lunch. The only thing I noticed was that Grandma would never come round to the house while Paul was there. She didn't like him at all. My dad didn't like him either. I still saw Dad every week and on those days it was a welcome contrast to the chaos with my mum. He wasn't happy leaving me at the mercy of Mum and her boyfriend but he was in a difficult situation, being in a new relationship and trying to keep contact with me.

Just when we were starting to think Paul had changed his ways, though, his old life came back with a vengeance.

Paul was in the house when there was a knock at the door down on the street below. We had a main door on ground level but all our rooms were up the stairs on the first floor. Mum looked out of the window.

A man called up: 'Is Paul there?'

Mum looked to Paul, who shook his head.

'He's not here,' Mum shouted down.

The man said something else but Mum couldn't make out what. She went down to tell him she didn't know when he'd be back. When she opened the door about twenty men carrying crowbars and other weapons barged past her. I was sitting at the top of the stairs and I screamed as they bulldozed their way up. They rushed into the flat and although Paul was hiding they found him instantly. From the noises coming from the bedroom they absolutely battered him. Mum ran up and I could hear her trying to pull them off her boyfriend, yelling at them to stop. I sat rooted to the spot, crying and shaking with fear, just wishing it would stop. Almost as fast as they arrived they were gone, piling down the stairs and into the street.

As the last man left, he turned to my mum, who was standing at the top of the stairs, and said: 'Sorry, Mandy.'

Mum took Paul to hospital. He had wounds all over his body. I heard Mum say it was a drug gang, obviously unhappy at something he had done. They were here to teach him a lesson. Thankfully they didn't hurt Mum. Paul's injuries were so severe he was in hospital for days.

That incident seemed to be a wake-up call for Paul, because when he came home things calmed down for a bit. They had the occasional row but it wasn't as bad as before. They actually seemed to be getting on, so much in fact that Mum told me that she and Paul were going to get married. Mum said it would be a chance for us to be a proper family. And as I was going to be her bridesmaid, it was an excuse to dress up. I could see in Mum's face that she was really excited. She and my dad hadn't married. She'd fallen pregnant after they'd been together for a year and having a baby had changed everything for them.

In the build-up to the big day, Mum showed me the pink dress she was going to wear. Despite all her problems, Mum was a beautiful woman, petite and curvy. She had dyed her natural fair hair black and styled it short and slick, like one of her idols, Lisa Stansfield. She even had the singer's black beauty spot on her cheek. My dress was also pink and matched hers. Paul had a new suit for the occasion. It was funny seeing us all dressed up.

They tied the knot in the local registry office. My grandma wasn't there, as she still couldn't stand Paul, but Auntie Marie and Uncle William came, along with Paul's brother and a couple of their friends.

It was all over quickly and when we came outside Marie threw confetti over us all. We went to a pub for a little celebration. It was a fun day. I don't think I'd ever seen my mum look so happy. If this was a sign of things to come, I liked the fact they got married.

My name changed to Jade Harries. Maybe Mum was right. We could be a proper, normal family.

Mum shouted less and didn't hit me as much and Paul didn't feel the need to hurt me either. In quieter moments Mum showed me how to draw. She took her time to teach me how to draw eyes and explained the distance between them and the nose and mouth. For birthdays and Christmas all I wanted was art supplies. Dad used to take me to Woolworths and spend £30 on paper, pens, charcoal pencils and stationery, and I couldn't wait to try them out. Mum could turn her hand to drawing anyone, like Elvis and Alanis Morissette, and her black-and-white sketches of the singers she really loved, like Madonna and Lisa

Stansfield, were on display around the house. She loved listening to music and I got my taste from her. I was into Texas and Gabrielle and more mature artists rather than a lot of the young poppy stuff that most children of my age liked. For the first time it felt like we were forming a bond.

Paul even managed to get in Grandma's good books. A film crew had turned up in our town to film an episode of *A Touch of Frost*, the drama series starring David Jason. They were looking for extras so Paul went along and landed a part as a policeman, ironically. When the episode aired we all sat down to watch it. It was funny seeing him on the small screen. Grandma was a huge fan of the programme so she was thrilled that she could go around telling people her son-in-law was in it. She was even happier when Paul used the money he got from it to paint her kitchen and kit it out with a new microwave and toaster. She softened her opinion of him, for a little while at least.

There were times when Paul did try to be a normal dad. He taught me to ride a bike that my real dad had got me. He also came home one day with a little Labrador puppy. Someone had rescued it and he thought I would like it. He was right. I loved it. We only had it for a week, though. I was out with it on my bike when it got caught under the wheels. It was yelping and although I tried to help it and it was okay, Mum wasn't happy and took it as a sign we shouldn't have a pet. We had to take it to the animal rescue centre. I was heartbroken. On the whole, though, we were getting on okay as a family.

But just when things were looking up, it all kicked off again – and this time it was worse than ever.

Chapter 3

'Come on,' Mum said. 'Quickly, it'll be fun. But you need to come now.'

Why was she whispering when we were the only people in the house? That's what I didn't understand. I followed her lead, though. She'd taken the quilt from my bed and laid it on the floor of the Wendy house in my room.

'Come on. Now!'

I climbed in to find her curled on the floor. I lay down next to her and she wrapped an arm around me and pulled the quilt over.

'Now stay quiet. Whatever happens. Not a sound, eh?'

I nodded and cuddled tightly into her. Although I was only four years old, it was so rare to have cuddle time with Mum I would gladly stay like this all night. Whatever game she was playing, it was a nice one.

Then I heard it. The noise from downstairs. Someone was entering the house. Mum moved her hand up to my mouth. I could feel my heart thumping as I heard the unmistakable sound of footsteps climbing the stairs. They could only belong to one person.

Paul had gone back to his old ways and when Mum found out he was back on drugs, she told him to leave. He hadn't taken it well. He kept trying to get back into the house to convince her to take him back – and worse, we suspected he was stealing things.

Obviously Mum didn't want to talk to him and didn't want him to know she was even in the house. Was she scared what he might do? I became scared too. Now I knew what was happening. He was coming for us. And Mum did not want him to find us.

He was taking his time, pausing every couple of steps. I concentrated really hard on not making a sound. But the more I concentrated the more scared I was that something would come out. Could he hear me breathing? Could he hear my heart beating? I could feel Mum's heart pounding against my back. Her breathing was quick, and in my ear it sounded like the wind blowing. Was it so loud he could hear?

He was at the top of the stairs now and I heard the creak of the kitchen door. There were a few steps and then I heard him entering the living room. Then it was Mum's room. It would be my room next.

Even though I was expecting it, my heart jumped when I realised he was in my room. I closed my eyes tight shut. Mum's grip hardened around me.

Please don't look inside, please don't look inside.

He seemed to stand there for an age. Was he even there at all? Had I imagined the whole thing?

Then I heard a floorboard creak and I wanted to scream with fear. This was real, very real.

More footsteps. They were quicker this time – and louder. They were going down the stairs, with no attempt to be quiet. The door opened and shut. We were alone again. He hadn't found what he was looking for.

I felt Mum's embrace loosen. I tried to turn and was about to say something when she whispered: 'Shhh! Not yet.'

We lay there for while longer. I was itching to get up. He was gone, surely we could move now? Mum wanted to make sure. For what seemed like twenty minutes we lay there before she climbed out of the Wendy house slowly and tiptoed to the door. I peeked out and saw her tentatively look out onto the landing. She held out a hand. Wait there. I heard her retrace the steps I'd just heard, flitting from room to room. Then she was back in the doorway.

'You can come out now.'

We'd got away with it … but it was only temporary respite and it wasn't long before Paul was back and causing more mayhem. Sometimes I witnessed the violence. All I could do was find somewhere to cower until it was over. There were other times when the only signs that trouble had started again were the repercussions and how they affected our lives.

The police had got involved and they believed Mum was in such danger from Paul they installed an alarm in the house. At night, when Mum set the alarm it meant no doors or windows could be opened. We just sat in the living room and had to be quiet. The TV was on mute with the subtitles on. One night Mum was too scared to go to bed so she said I could stay up late with her. At first it was exciting and it felt special to be getting quality time with my mum, but after a little while my eyes started to get heavy and all I wanted was my bed.

'Not yet,' Mum whispered. 'Stay awake a little longer.'

I must have dozed off because it was 2 a.m. and we still hadn't gone to bed. I was about to ask Mum again but suddenly there was a bang. Someone was trying to get in the kitchen window. A split second later the alarm went off. I jumped out of my skin. It was so loud I was sure it must have burst my eardrum.

Mum grabbed me and we ran down the stairs to the front door and straight out into the street. I was in my bare feet and Mum picked me up and started running. The screeching of the alarm rang in my ears. In the quiet of the night it seemed ten times louder than any car or house alarm. I was so scared I just clung on to her and she ran, heaving for breath. I knew something bad was going to happen if he caught us.

We must have run for about twenty minutes. Mum couldn't carry me anymore so she put me down and I had to run with her. My feet hardly touched the ground as we raced through the streets. Eventually Mum saw a phone box and pushed me inside. She called the police and we waited there until they came to get us.

We didn't speak much. Mum kept looking out the windows, on all sides. It was the first time I'd seen her scared. Paul must have threatened her and the threats must have been serious enough for the police to be involved. It was only then my feet started to hurt and I realised how cold I was. I was so grateful to see the police car. They told us they'd searched for Paul and had found him in a shed in a neighbouring back garden. As they had him in custody it was safe for us to go back to the house. There were people at their windows and out on the street to see what the fuss was about.

Given how scared my mum was that night she must have realised that their relationship was toxic but she just couldn't help herself. There were times she wanted to be away from him and there were times she wanted him back.

When I next saw my dad I came back and told Mum I wanted to move in with him.

'He has just got you to say that,' she said.

'No,' I said. 'I just want to be with my dad.' It was true. I liked being with him. It was a nicer experience, without the constant threat of violence or fear.

My mum was adamant I could not go to my dad. I had no choice. I had to live with her – whatever the consequences. And for me, those consequences were brutal. Not being with Paul brought out the worst in Mum.

Rarely did I know what would set her off. One minute she'd be okay and the next she was screaming. So even though Paul had hurt me and we'd had to hide and flee from the house to get away from him, I begged Mum to take him back. I clung to the memories of the times when things were calmer.

Before too long she did take him back and, just like before when they first got married, everything was rosy. Mum told me she was expecting a baby. We'd be a proper little family. In August 1993, nearly two months after my fifth birthday and shortly before I started school, she gave birth to a boy, Jack. It was exciting to have a baby brother. Everyone doted on him, including me. Mum encouraged me to call Paul 'Dad', so I did, but he would never replace my real dad.

In just a few short months, though, all thoughts that we could be a normal family went out the window. Mum and Paul started fighting again and now when they rowed it turned violent. When I heard them screaming at each other I went to my room and put my hands over my ears, but it was no use. I could still hear them. I crawled into my Wendy house, pulled my duvet in with me and curled up, wrapping the quilt over my head in a bid to block it out. Still I could hear them yelling. It was often like this. Mum would kick off about something and Paul would yell back at her. That was my cue to take myself off until it eventually calmed down.

I was getting good at spotting the signs that it was about to kick off. Maybe Paul hadn't been home for a couple of days, or maybe when he did show up he looked and smelled funny. Mum would then accuse him of being up to his old tricks again.

When I felt the house shake I knew Paul had stormed out. I wouldn't see him for a few weeks. It was obvious then that my mother had broken up with him. After a few weeks Paul would come around being all nice and winning over my mother. She was always glad to see him back. I could tell she loved him. Often when Paul returned he'd have a load of presents, like a new DVD player or a stereo or a bike for me. He'd make lots of promises about changing and how he meant it this time.

Sometimes I would be glad to see him back because although they shouted at each other a lot and threw things at each other, when he wasn't here it was worse. Mum missed him and cried a lot. On top of that she was struggling with being a single parent and trying to raise two young children. She was angry all the time and took her fury out on me. She'd hit me for nothing, scream at me over the tiniest thing and I'd never know what would set her off next time.

We never seemed to have enough money for even the basics, like food, and everything was a struggle. So many times everything got too much for her and she would erupt.

One day she came at me, seemingly for no reason. Before I could react she grabbed me by the hair and yanked me across the floor. She lashed out, catching me on the eye. I screamed in pain and cried for her to stop. It was only then she calmed down and burst into tears.

Then one morning I woke up and went to go out of my bedroom. The door was locked from the outside. I banged the door to get out and called: 'Mum!'

After a moment, Mum let me out. She didn't say a word. I didn't know what I had done to upset her but she seemed in a mood. I went into the living room and heard Mum going into the kitchen. The next thing she came into the room wielding a wooden mop handle and started hitting me with it. I screamed. She caught me on the shin and I've never felt pain like it. It felt like the bottom of my leg had been split open. I was bleeding and it was only then I saw there was a nail at the bottom of the handle. It had gone straight into my leg.

I was so shocked at the sudden violence, I could barely even cry. I was gulping a huge lungful of air with each breath. Only when Mum saw how badly she'd hurt me did she calm down and act all apologetic. She took me to hospital to get the wound seen to. I couldn't believe she had come at me like that. It was like she was possessed.

Mum had been known to social services ever since she was younger and now they became involved. A social worker came round and spoke to her about her behaviour but, despite what she'd put me through, when they spoke to me I clammed up. Mum might have been horrible to me but I didn't want anything to happen to her. I didn't know what to say. I just wanted her to be happy.

Going to school should have been an exciting time for me, a chance to make new friends and leave the troubles of home behind for a few hours a day, but it just wasn't like that at all. The school was very much involved with Mum and me and social services. From as far back as I can remember the teachers always wanted to know what was going on at home. I just wanted to fit in and not have anyone make a fuss, but they used to take me into a different room and question me. I wouldn't speak because I knew what they were trying to do. There were so many questions: 'Have you eaten today?' 'What's your mum made you?' 'Is your dad at home just now?'

I knew not to speak to anyone because I thought it would get my mum into trouble. I just used to mumble some answers or try to tell them what I thought they wanted to hear. I had to protect my mum, everyone was questioning me and I was defensive all the time. Every time I was asked a question I thought, 'What are you asking me that for?' I was guarded and the teachers probably thought I was an angry little child.

When I got home Mum would hit me with even more questions: 'What's happened? What were they asking you? What did you tell them?'

Or she'd send me to school in the morning, saying, 'Don't tell them that Paul is here.'

I felt loyalty to my mum and I was desperate to please her so I did what she said. It was just very stressful. Everywhere I turned there were adults involved in my life. School wasn't pleasurable. There were no fun times that I can remember.

I didn't feel like a normal child. I looked at everyone else playing in the playground, looking as though they didn't have a care in the world, and I wondered why I couldn't be like that. Why did I have to be the one with the parents who fought all the time?

I was always aware that I couldn't relax and just be a child. There was constant embarrassment as well. Children know when someone is being treated differently so they eyed me suspiciously. Parents gossip among themselves and to their children, and one or two kids said things about my mum. As a result I didn't form the same friendships with other children that normal kids do. I just remember feeling embarrassment from a young age. I saw some classmates being friendly with the teacher but I never had a normal relationship with any of the adults. It was like everyone interrogated me. They all wanted to know something.

The only friend I had at school was a girl called Ellie. She was the daughter of one of Mum's friends who lived nearby. We got up to mischief together. We found some black shoe polish and wrote our full names on the toilet door. The teachers called us out of class and asked why we'd done it. We swore blind it wasn't us, even when they pointed out we'd written our own names. They made us wipe it off. We got into trouble but it was about the best fun I had at school.

I had a better time playing in the street near our house. I used to play with a boy called Luke, the son of another of Mum's friends. We hung out in each other's houses and watched *Batman* together. I was a tomboy and preferred hanging out with Luke to the girls that lived locally. I was obsessed with Bruce Lee as a child. I watched all his films and ran around doing his moves and fighting with the boys on the street. At five and six I never wanted to wear a top and preferred to run around like the boys. My mum was always telling me to put some clothes on. She tried to make me more demure by enrolling me in ballet lessons. I loved it, but after watching *Dirty Dancing* with my mum I was more interested in learning Latin dance. I was captivated by the close, sultry, provocative form of dancing in the movie, especially during the 'Love Man' scene, and I said to Mum, 'I want to do that.'

She said, 'Absolutely not.'

Aside from Bruce Lee and *Batman*, I also loved *Knight Rider*. That was a Sunday night thing in our house and one of my fondest memories – when they weren't kicking off – was having Sunday dinner, which Mum would prepare, and then sitting down to watch it with Mum and Paul. These were rare moments of joy.

Largely, though, I just felt like I was treated differently at home, as well as at school. My brother had grown into boisterous toddler. He was hyperactive but he was a mummy's boy. He'd get into trouble for being hyper but Mum never hit him like she hit me. She might tap his legs or lightly scold him if he misbehaved, the normal reprimanding of a child. It wasn't over the top. She would sit him on the stairs until he calmed down.

With me, though, she continued to lash out. It wasn't fair.

Our home situation became an even greater challenge for Mum when, out of the blue, in August 1995, when I was seven, she discovered she was pregnant again. She didn't even know she was expecting. She hadn't put on any weight and two weeks after Jack's second birthday she ended up in hospital and gave birth to a little girl. It was a shock to everyone.

Mum said I could choose what to call her so I said I wanted to name her after my best friend Ellie.

'How about we call her Ellen but you can call her Ellie if you like?'

That's what happened. When Mum came home with her it was quickly apparent that she hadn't bonded with Ellie in the same way she had with Jack or me. Not knowing she was pregnant meant she hadn't had time to get used to the idea. Now Mum, who was still only 24 and hadn't been coping for years, had three young children to look after.

Ellie was just a baby, so Mum wouldn't take her anger out on her, but I could see there wasn't much affection. I felt the need to mother Ellie myself, to make up for it. I knew I had to look out for my brother and sister. The trouble was, who was looking out for me?

Chapter 4

I was in the house playing when I realised there was banging coming from outside. It was December 1995, four months after Ellen was born. Mum had gone out, leaving the three of us in the house with Paul. I could hear her shouting outside. What was going on? Why wasn't she in the house?

'Jade!' Paul shouted. 'Get Jack and Ellen. Come into the living room.'

There was a lot of banging and movement of furniture coming from inside. I did as I was told, got my siblings and we made our way tentatively into the living room. The room was in semi-darkness because the curtains were drawn but we could still see the place was a mess. Paul had moved furniture about. There were chairs overturned, ornaments knocked over and stuff everywhere. Paul looked mad, like his face was about to burst. He was jumping about frantically and kept going to the window, pulling back the curtains and shouting down to the street. I could hear my mum screaming, 'Don't hurt the kids!'

Once we were inside he shut the door and moved the sofa and other bits and pieces over to barricade us in. He hauled the table nearer to the window. A picture frame got knocked off the wall and smashed on the floor.

My brother and sister were scared, their lips trembling. I tried to reassure them but I was frightened too.

'What's going on?' I said, my voice shaking.

'Come here!' He grabbed me hard by the wrist and hauled me to the window. He was hurting me so I tried to do what he wanted, whatever that was. He pulled me up and made me sit on the table. He pulled back the curtains and I blinked at the sudden exposure to the light. When my eyes adjusted I looked below and could see Mum there on the street. She was banging on the door. The neighbours were out watching the unfolding drama.

'Here's Jade! She's fine.' Paul was manic. Now there was light in the room I could see his eyes were like pinpricks. I knew what that meant. He was back on drugs. 'Tell your mum you're fine.'

'I'm okay, Mum,' I called. 'So are Jack and Ellen.'

'Let me in, Paul, for God's sake! What are you doing?'

'Just go and get the bloody money!' Paul shouted, still gripping me by the wrist so tightly I could feel my skin burn.

I didn't know how we'd got to this situation but it was obvious he wanted Mum to get him money for drugs. They shouted at each other, Jack and Ellen started crying. It was chaos. I wanted to go and cuddle them but I couldn't move.

'Please let me check they're okay,' I said, starting to well up.

Without warning he yanked the curtains shut again and pushed me down from the table. He shoved me onto the carpet and I screamed in agony. I could feel my face being cut to shreds. I couldn't work out what was happening. Then I realised. My head had gone right into the broken picture frame. I got up from the floor and put my hands to my face. They were covered in blood that was now pouring down my face. Paul was still shouting. Amid the chaos I could hear Mum yell that she was away to get the money. She was saying something about the police. Were they outside or on their way? We were still barricaded in the darkness. I was crying, trying to stem the bleeding. Paul shouted at us all to stop crying, which only made us sob even more.

It must only have been a few minutes but it seemed like an eternity that we were trapped in there, Paul screaming out the window to anyone who would listen. Mum then came back. I could hear her shouting that she'd got the money.

'Put it through the letterbox,' Paul yelled.

Mum did so. Paul moved the furniture away from the door and ran downstairs. I heard the back door open and he must have fled, as I didn't hear him anymore.

'Jade, you need to let me in,' Mum shouted.

I checked Jack and Ellen were okay and then ran downstairs and opened the front door. Mum was horrified at the cuts to my face. She comforted my brother and sister and they eventually calmed down. We went to hospital and although I didn't need stitches, I had several bad scars.

It was December 1995 and Paul went missing for a few days after that. Mum said that was the final straw. In the weeks leading up to him effectively holding us hostage Paul had been taking heroin again. That had led to them rowing once more, and their arguments often turning violent. It was when Mum refused to cash in her benefit money to get him more drugs that he'd barricaded us in. In the aftermath of that day Paul was still in and out of our lives until eventually, after Mum spoke to social workers, it was decided that, for all of our safety, we move temporarily to a women's refuge.

'We'll be safe there,' Mum said.

I had no choice but to go along with it. I thought if it made Mum a little happier then it could be a good thing. I honestly think at times Mum wanted away from Paul and away from the drugs, the violence. She despised drugs and had never even smoked a cigarette at this stage of her life. I think she really believed this was a fresh start for her and her children. The refuge was not far from where we lived. We had a self-contained apartment with a kitchenette and bathroom, and there was a communal living room. Other children were staying there at the same time, who were, like us, fleeing their mothers' violent partners. There was a manager who also lived in the quarters and no one was allowed in who wasn't authorised. Mum could go out as normal but you weren't allowed friends over and we couldn't have family visit. It was all about our protection.

We were to be there for a few weeks, which meant we'd be spending Christmas in there. Mum told us not to worry, that Father Christmas would know where to find us. I felt sad because it wasn't going to be the same. Like all kids I looked forward to Christmas. Mum always made a big deal of it and it was one of the few days a year when nice things happened. We would go to the pub where Mum worked, which opened for a few hours in the afternoon. Grandma would be there, and Marie and William and the regulars made a fuss of us and gave us money. There was always a lovely atmosphere. At our house, normally I would be the one to get up at 5 a.m. One year I was convinced I looked out of the window and saw Father Christmas leaving on his sleigh. Dad would give his gifts to Mum beforehand so we had them to open as well. Previously, even though

Jack was not his child, he made sure he always put a gift in for him. Now Ellie was here too I was sure he'd do the same but I wouldn't see him until after Christmas.

Dad was always buying me a new bike because although Paul had taught me how to ride it he used to steal them to sell for drugs. The bikes were usually kept in a laundry room off the kitchen and one time we came home from shopping and my bike was gone. The small window in the room was open. Paul claimed someone must have opened the window, climbed in and taken the bike, but there was no way the bike would have fitted through the window. Mum shouted at him to get the bike back. He never did, so Dad would have to buy a new one. He said to Mum that if he bought a new one it would stay at his house because he didn't trust Paul.

That was the legacy of living with a lying, thieving drug dealer. And now another consequence was that we were spending Christmas in a refuge. It was like we were being punished for something, yet we had done nothing wrong.

Throughout this time I had more meetings with social workers and an educational psychologist. My school said I had a lot of problems. Once again, though, I refused to cooperate with an adult asking me questions. I couldn't see how any good would come of it. I had bruises on my face, not just caused by the scarring from Paul's violence. Mum was still hitting me when she became angry, which was a lot.

I never knew what would set her off. And it was terrifying how violent she became. Once when she was yelling at me I ran out of the room. She was still screaming so I stuck my head back around the door. Something hit me full in the face. It was a jug Mum had thrown.

On another occasion she came into my bedroom and pounced on me, pinning me down on the bed. I tried to shout and scream but the air was knocked out of me. I was struggling to find my breath. She grabbed my pillow and put it over my face. I panicked even more, flaying my arms and legs, trying to do anything to get her off. What was happening? Was she actually trying to kill me? What had I done?

Suddenly she let go and lifted the pillow off my face. I gasped for breath and leapt to my feet, in case she came for me again. She just put the pillow down and without saying a word walked out of the room like nothing had happened. I sat on the floor, my heart thumping, racing, trying to work out what had just happened – and why.

Even thinking about that incident now upsets me because the only question that runs through my head is: how could someone hurt a child that way? Her own child. How could a mother have that much hate in her body?

Life was pretty miserable in the women's refuge. Mum was in such a foul mood a lot of the time that I tried to keep out of her way as much as possible.

Sometimes I used to go downstairs and sit in the manager's office and watch soaps with her on TV because I didn't want to be with my mum. Anything was better than being in our apartment, not knowing when she was going to kick off.

She promised the social workers that she had split from Paul for good, but he still had control over her, even when they weren't physically together. Mum told me Paul was in prison – for what I didn't know, but most likely it was for drug offences. He was in Strangeways Prison, in Manchester, which wasn't that far away from us.

When we moved out of the refuge into another flat, Mum made plans to go and see him. It wasn't enough to just go and visit him, however. He made specific demands of her – and even though she was anti-drugs, and even though she knew how violent he had been towards us, it was like she couldn't say no. She was completely under his control.

Jack was then two and still in nappies. The prison guards patted me down but they never used to search small children so Mum hid drugs inside Jack's nappies. Even though there were cameras everywhere, Paul was allowed to have Jack on his lap. Mum had cut the lining of the nappy and stuffed the drugs into where the soft filling of the nappy would be. Paul would discreetly work his fingers inside and fiddle around until he had removed the package.

Another ruse she employed was to cut holes inside her pockets and secure wraps to her knickers and once she was inside the visiting hall she'd work the packet loose and give it to him. I knew all this because Mum did it in front of me before we went to see him. One of the neighbours came over and helped her. Paul was ordering her to do it and she was unable to say no. She was completely at his mercy.

Throughout this time I wasn't at school and it was hard to stay in touch with the few friends I had made. From the moment we had entered the women's refuge it was the beginning of a period where we seemed to be constantly on the move. We moved from temporary flats to another refuge to homeless hostels and other properties in Greater Manchester and the surrounding area.

We spent a second Christmas in a women's refuge. This time was even bleaker than the last. Mum was in a foul mood. As usual, we had no idea what had set her off but she was determined to punish us for something. On Christmas morning she tried to say Father Christmas hadn't been but I saw the curtains in the communal living area were bulging out and spied some bags of presents behind them. I don't know what we'd done wrong but she refused to give them to us until much later that night. By then the fun times we'd had on Christmas Days in the past were distant memories.

It was a chaotic way to live. We only had a few belongings so life was a regular change of clothes, beds and other furniture. I soon learned not to become attached to my belongings as, almost without warning, we would be moving again and I'd never see certain things again.

Social services gave Mum grants to kit us out in new clothes. She started to order through catalogues. Sometimes a package of new clothes arrived. Mum would then get on the phone and say it hadn't been delivered. They'd send out the same again and Mum sold the extra clothes on. They just used to leave the parcels outside the door so there was no way of them knowing if we'd received them or not. She did this with trainers, coats, everything.

Occasionally I would start at a new school but in a matter of weeks we'd move again and I'd have to begin all over again. I missed out on a lot of education. And at each school the process was the same. Teachers would interrogate me about my home life and I would clam up. I went to at least five or six schools over two years and as a result not only was it impossible to make lasting friendships but I felt victimised and bullied, forever the new girl with no fixed abode. Despite the challenging circumstances I tried to work hard in class, but just when I'd feel I was catching up we'd move once more and I had to start from scratch.

When Paul was nearing his release, social workers were asking Mum what she intended to do. They knew she was writing to him in prison and they were warning her not to get back together with him or she might risk losing her children. There were times during this period when we were put into respite care. It was obvious to everyone that she wasn't coping but temporary care seemed to be the best they could come up with. I have vague memories of being placed with a kind older woman for a week. It was bliss to be out of the chaos with Mum. Jack and Ellen were put somewhere else. Despite Mum's anger towards me she missed me when I wasn't there and always wanted me back – even before she got Jack and Ellen. I remember there was one time when Jack spent a short time in a seaside town, perhaps to give Mum some respite. We had to visit social services there but for whatever reason Mum was not happy and started kicking off.

'Well, keep Jack then,' she said, leaving him on a desk in social services and taking me with her. I was thinking, 'You can't leave him there.'

The social workers were yelling at her to come back but it looked like she was being serious. Eventually she calmed down enough to see sense and went back to get him. I think her point was that she didn't have the money to look after all three of us and unless they helped her she had no option but to leave one of us with them.

There was another time when we were in Blackpool because Mum took Ellen to see social services. My real dad had family nearby and we saw them at the same time. I remember being in the arcades, playing the 2p machines and the coin fountains.

Maybe Mum's antics with social services had some effect because when I was around eight years old we moved to a new home in a neighbouring county. Paul was still not around. From what I could gather he was in prison and had moved from Strangeways to another one in Lancaster, prior to his release.

For a brief period we had some sort of stability. Uncle William lived with us and Mum took on a couple of jobs in pubs to earn some extra money. Grandma visited us and on some level it felt a little like it had been in the very early days. However, being with Mum meant there was always some sense of disruption. She spent so much time at one of the pubs we often stayed there with her and divided our time between there and the house.

The sad thing for me was that since our life had become nomadic, contact with my real dad had become less frequent. By the time we moved, that contact was in danger of completely breaking down. Mum was being difficult and not making it easy for us to see each other. It didn't help when I was put into respite care, like I was when Mum decided to go on holiday with William and a man from the pub. They were going to Tenerife. We might not have been going with her but at least we got a holiday from Mum's erratic behaviour. Even with the holiday she

managed to create drama because she lost her passport in the run-up.

She had not been back long when, in March 1996,
while I was still seven, there was yet another emergency
when Mum put the chip pan on but then nipped next
door to a neighbour's house. She hadn't taken a key and
when the door closed behind her she was locked out. I
was outside playing but Ellen was trapped inside in her
bedroom. While one neighbour called the fire brigade
a couple of others attempted to climb up a pipe to get
into the top bedroom window. They didn't manage it
and it took the firefighters to break into the house to
make sure Ellen was okay. She wasn't hurt, and apart
from some smoke the house wasn't damaged, but it was
a close call.

Once again, no sooner had we started to get used to
our new surroundings than we were on the move again,
this time to an old mill town not far from our first
home.

Social services resumed contact with my dad, which
I was extremely pleased about but Mum wasn't happy.
We met in a contact centre in the town and Mum
started screaming at me to tell her where my dad lived
– as she wanted money from him. It spilled out into the
street and she was still yelling at me in front of stunned
passers-by. Social workers were very much involved in
our lives and they warned Mum again about resuming
contact with Paul. He was now out of prison and if he

tried to come back and live with us they believed we were in grave danger of further assaults. Mum told them what they wanted to hear. I didn't know what to think. All I wanted was my old mum back, the one who used to show me how to draw and sang with me to her favourite music. But that mum was just a distant memory – and in her place was a troubled soul who was losing what last grip she had on reality.

And I would be the one to suffer most as a consequence.

Chapter 5

My heart thumped as I handed over the book. I was sure my face screamed guilty. I could feel everyone's eyes on me.

'You'll be fine, Jade. Just act natural,' Mum had said. This was important to her. I couldn't let her down. I wanted to please her, wanted her to be proud of me. But if this was such a good idea – why did it feel so wrong?

The woman behind the post office counter took the giro book. She glanced at the page and then at me. I tried to smile, hoping my face said, 'Nothing to see here. Just go about your business and process it as normal.'

She looked again at the book. She must know. This was a stupid idea. I was going to get caught.

'Mum not with you today?'

'No,' I said. 'Not feeling well.'

'That's a shame. Lot of bugs about.'

I nodded and had a glance around to see if anyone was coming towards me, like a guard of some kind. It looked fairly normal. I turned back to the woman who had a stamp out, thumped it on the book and counted out the cash. She handed it to me. I stuffed it into a pocket and got out of there as fast as I could to where Mum was waiting outside.

'Okay?'

I showed her the bundle.

'That's my girl.'

She was happy. I'd done well. That was the best I could hope for. After that success, she tried it more often. Mum and a neighbour had worked out the way to defraud the benefits system. Using her skills as an artist she meticulously cut out tiny bits of paper and using a fountain pen wrote a date and carefully stuck it into the giro book. On Tuesdays she got her money as usual, then she sent me in with the doctored book to make her claim again. Both she and the neighbour were at it.

After the success of that first time they were keen to keep trying. When I went back the following week I felt more confident. Mum was right. It was easy. I took in the book, handed it over, the teller made a cursory glance at the book and the date, stamped it and handed over the cash. Looking back, it was quite entrepreneurial but there was also something very wrong about getting an eight-year-old girl to carry out your benefit fraud.

For several weeks we tried it and every time it worked. I started to get a bit bolder and thought nothing of going into the post office and queuing with all the adults. That was until the time when the woman paused longer than normal over the book. She studied the slip.

'Who are you here with?' she said. There was no smile. No small talk. She looked at me with a deadly serious expression on her face. I started to burn up. She shook her head. 'No.'

I turned and ran out of the post office. Mum was outside as normal and now I was scared to tell her I'd got turned away. I was relieved that at least we only got told no. It could have been much worse. Mum was cross though. She was relying on that money. She never seemed to have enough. It would take me some time to work out why.

Early on in our new home it was clear we faced a new type of threat. We were living in quite a large house, over three levels. The first inkling I got was when someone smashed a downstairs window. A couple of days later another was put in. Mum got anxious. She couldn't settle and at night, once she'd put Jack and Ellen to bed, she begged me to stay up with her.

'Just sit with me, Jade. It will be fun, just me and you.'

It was like the times when she was worried Paul was going to hurt us. Just as then, I wanted to be with

54

her, because at night-time she wasn't as angry, just agitated. I stayed up as late as I could but I got so tired. She put the telly on but got up constantly to see if someone was coming to the house. She was living on her nerves.

'I think people are looking for your dad,' she said, referring to Paul. He hadn't been at the house but when they found out who my mum was they took an interest in her. They didn't know that she hadn't seen him for years but they knew he had the name Harries and put two and two together. Jack and Ellen were his kids. If Paul was in hiding from the drug gangs he used to associate with, or if rivals were out for revenge over some dodgy deal and if they couldn't get Paul, then we were the next best thing. Whatever Paul had done to make someone that angry we could only guess, but they were taking it out on us.

I don't think Mum really knew who was targeting us. We had seen a gang exact its violent revenge on Paul before when men attacked him with crowbars so she knew what this type of people were capable of. As the weeks dragged on she got increasingly agitated. She was getting thinner as well. She stopped eating and wasn't cooking proper meals for us. Still she sat up late but sometimes, even though she stopped me from falling asleep, she'd nod off on the sofa. She then woke up angry that she'd dozed off. She vowed to do something about it and started taking speed to keep her awake.

She'd go for days without sleeping and it made her irritable and spaced out.

Then I began noticing the telltale signs I'd seen in Paul when he was on drugs. Her pupils went really small and the weight fell off her. No longer was she the curvy, vivacious mother I once knew, but a gaunt, skinny figure whose clothes hung off her and skin sagged. I suspected she was taking heroin – the same drug Paul was addicted to – to help her sleep after being strung out for several days on the trot.

That's when things really unravelled.

Mum just wasn't looking after us. She was paranoid someone was going to turn up – whether it was Paul or someone out to get him. She had social services in the background warning her not to make contact with Paul or she'd lose us for good. She was running out of money and was so strung out she failed in her duties as a mother.

None of us were going to school or nursery. We didn't have proper bedding, our clothes were filthy and there was no food in the house. When I think back to the times when social workers quizzed me in the past about whether I was eating properly, at that point it was fine. Mum would prepare breakfast for us, mostly cornflakes, we'd get dinners at school and she'd cook a tea for us. Social workers used to give her food vouchers. Now, though, we had nothing – or if Mum was getting money or vouchers they weren't being used to feed us. Often I was starving but I felt my priority was to feed my brother and sister. Mum simply wasn't eating, but we had to.

Both Jack and Ellen were fairly easy to cater for. He was obsessed with jam on toast so I kept making that for him, or I made sure he had rusks so he could eat them as a biscuit or I poured milk on them to make porridge. I bought Smarties but Jack didn't like the orange ones so I used to pick them out before giving them to him. Ellen was still on a bottle of milk so I just had to make sure I had enough to keep her filled up. I felt an enormous amount of pressure as the eldest to look after them, especially Ellen, as I knew Mum had never bonded with her.

Mum received milk tokens with her giro, which you could exchange in the local store for bread and milk up to that value. I would go to get it but sometimes didn't have enough tokens to make up the full amount. I said to the shopkeeper Mum would drop the rest off when she got her giro.

Previously Mum paid that bill, as it was our local shop, but he said, 'Your mum hasn't been in. Is she avoiding me? She needs to settle up.'

I just shrugged and said I'd tell her. What else could I do? I felt like I was the adult in our house. If the milk tokens were no longer an option I had to find other ways to feed us.

Our local doctor's surgery had a coffee vending machine that served hot chocolate. I went in and told the receptionists we were hungry. They gave me hot chocolates and lollies. That prompted some action because a health visitor came to the house to check on our wellbeing. She was shocked to see us eating the last of some Weetabix out of one dirty saucepan. It was the only food we had left. The milk in the fridge had long since gone off, curdled and separated. It was another example of someone in a position of responsibility seeing for themselves the conditions we had to put up with.

Social workers also came to the house to check up on Mum and seemed shocked by what they found. I wasn't sure if they believed me when I said there was no food in the house. They arranged for us to be given a food parcel.

The social workers did at least make some headway with the local school. They had expressed their dismay that none of us were going to school and one asked me when was the last time I had actually been. A meeting was arranged at the local school but Mum kept falling asleep in the headteacher's office, complaining that she hadn't slept for two weeks. I started school again but Mum hadn't sorted dinners so often I went hungry during the day until the arrangements had been made for me to eat. Mum had the food vouchers but hadn't given them to the school.

It was just a never-ending state of neglect, of which social services were routinely made aware. Neighbours complained when Mum locked us out of the house and they saw us stuck outside for hours. A bus driver got involved when he saw Ellen, who was then just turning three, wandering the streets. He kindly took her home and made sure she was okay.

Grandma rang them about her own daughter's negligence or cruelty. Amid everything else that was going on, Mum still routinely lost her rag with me. A couple of days before my tenth birthday, in June 1998, she came at me with a mad look in her eye. I was eating a Toffee Crisp chocolate bar and I got such a fright I nearly choked. She slapped me around the face and to avoid being hit further I jumped around a camp bed but smashed my eye on the metal frame. My eye immediately swelled and turned black and purple.

Mum panicked. 'Social services are going to take you off me and accuse me of hitting you when they see that.'

By the day of my birthday I was sporting a large, shining black eye. In previous years, Mum had made a big fuss of my special day, often taking us to McDonald's as a treat. I would remember this one, but for much different reasons. She didn't think she was responsible because technically she hadn't caused the bruise and the swollen eye, even though I had been running away from her initial slap.

An official from the council's housing department paid a visit the next day but Mum wouldn't let him in.

He called through the letterbox and saw me. He asked how I got the black eye.

'I fell and hit my head on the bed,' I said.

I don't think he believed me. Mum was in the background, listening and passing messages to me. He couldn't see her but I suspected he knew what was going on.

A council joiner then came to do some repairs and noticed Mum had locked Jack in the top bedroom. The door was shut and he was crying to get out. Neighbours complained again when they saw Jack running around outside without shoes on when Mum was supposed to be looking after him.

Social workers were now paying regular visits to the house, almost on a daily basis. One day we had been outside at a neighbour's house. It was the end of June and still warm but Jack just had a t-shirt on and boxer shorts and Ellen was in a pyjama top with no underwear. When they asked why we were outside dressed like that, Mum got really defensive and started shouting. One of the social workers mentioned that several neighbours had reported seeing us outside, unsupervised. Mum kicked off, yelling about 'interfering neighbours' and would get so angry the social workers cut short their meeting and left.

Mum's doctor prescribed her methadone to try to wean her off heroin and that brought about a change in her appearance, if not her attitude. Despite the lack of proper nutrition her weight ballooned and her skin became puffy. Being on methadone, however, was another accident waiting to happen. When next a social worker called – and Mum actually let her in the house – she found the methadone prescription sitting on top of the television in easy of reach of us children. She told Mum about the potential dangers but, as serious as it was, it was just another example of where Mum's priorities lay. She was more interested in drugs by then than our wellbeing.

In the weeks before the end of the school term, I did not attend school. Mum was just out of it for large parts of the day, after being up most of the night. I was exhausted too, through lack of food and running around after my brother and sister. I never saw caring for them as a chore. I doted on them and was only concerned about making sure they ate something, but it was extremely tiring. It was also near impossible to keep on top of everything.

I tried to get help by ringing the social services' emergency number, telling the person on the other end of the line that once again we had no food. A day later they delivered a food parcel. At last we were able to eat but all semblance of order had disappeared in the house. Mum was at the end of her tether and at times pleaded for Jack, who was still boisterous and difficult to discipline, to be taken into care. I couldn't watch over them all hours of the day and night, and for that reason it was almost inevitable when a neighbour saw Ellen outside the house, on a warm July night, at 3 a.m. wandering around with no clothes on. No harm came to her but if that wasn't a sign that Mum was completely failing in her duties I didn't know what was.

The reports were so frequent social workers did drive-bys of the house to see what was happening. I got to know their cars. The same two social workers regularly checked up on us. Only one of them I found warm. She was called Shona and she seemed to really sympathise with my situation. She visited sometime after my birthday when Mum was again giving me a hard time. Dad had given me a present for my birthday and had tried to help out the rest of the family by handing over a food hamper. Mum saw this as an opportunity and told me to ask my dad for money. Shona intervened and said it wasn't appropriate to ask me to do this. She gave Mum food vouchers instead, which seemed to calm her down.

The vouchers only provided temporary reprieve from our neglect, though. Before long the food would run out, there would be no money and once again we were at the mercy of social services. Their task was made doubly difficult when they asked to check what food we had and Mum once again refused to let them in the house. As they were leaving Mum rushed out with Ellen and left her on the doorstep, asking them to take her off her. When they refused and continued to their car, Mum picked Ellen up and lifted her onto the bonnet. They said they would look at a temporary solution.

Not long after, when Mum was kicking off at me again, I saw Shona's car drive by. I approached the car and asked her if I could be put into foster care.

'No, I can't do that. I'm sorry,' Shona said and drove off.

I was exhausted and heartbroken. I had always tried to protect Mum but now I was tired of her constant apologies for her violence. I was drained from trying to please her all the time, trying to win her love. I wanted my brother and sister to be looked after properly, bathed regularly and for them to sleep in a comfortable bed. I wanted them to be loved. I wanted someone to rescue us and I knew I didn't want to go back. I wanted to be given away. I didn't understand why social services wouldn't help. What was the point of them receiving all these reports and having meetings with us when they didn't seem to do anything? They just seemed to take notes and arrange countless visits.

Would anything be done?

I had no idea, but in the meantime I had no option but to go along with it. I tried to make the best of the situation, but just when I thought it could not get any worse I got a new shock.

I was in Mum's room, jumping on her bed, listening to Alanis Morissette, when the cupboard door clicked open. I jumped off and went to close it. Spying something inside, my nosiness got the better of me and I saw a blue and white sports bag. I knelt down and began to unzip it. Inside were several large shotguns and one small handgun. I couldn't believe what I was seeing. Whose were they? Why were they in our house?

Just then the bedroom door flung open and Mum was standing there.

'Don't go in there!' she yelled. Then she softened her tone and crouched down to hug me. She zipped up the bag and closed the door. I was almost as shocked by her change of attitude as I was to seeing the firearms. Was she relieved that there hadn't been an accident? We went downstairs and she immediately called someone on the phone.

I heard her tell whomever she was speaking to, 'Pick the bag up now. I can't have them around the children.'

The next time I was brave enough to peek inside the cupboard the bag was gone.

Mum might have had a narrow escape on that occasion. Next time she would not be so lucky.

Chapter 6

I woke with a start.

BANG!

It took me a moment to work out what I was hearing.

BANG! BANG!

It was coming from downstairs. The whole house was shaking. It sounded like we were under attack. There was an almighty crash and then shouting. We *were* under attack! Was this the moment Mum had feared? Had a drug gang come for us?

I jumped out of bed. It sounded like the whole house was being taken over. There were lots of men shouting and I could hear people crashing from room to room. I was terrified. I couldn't hear Mum. Then I saw who it was. The police. Dozens of them, it seemed, filling up the doorways and hall. They looked huge with their uniforms and gear. I didn't fully appreciate it at that moment but it was a drugs raid. I stood there bewildered as they crashed around me. One officer told me to go to the living room where I'd find Jack and Ellen. I went through and there were people everywhere. It was like an invasion. A female officer was there with a social worker I recognised. They crouched down to our level and spoke slowly and kindly, explaining that they were having to search the house and that we would be able to get dressed, gather some things and pack a rucksack because we would still be going to school as normal.

Then I saw Mum. She looked shocked and frantic, watching as the police went from room to room. They were tearing the place up, ripping cushions from the sofa and chairs and emptying drawers and anything that could be used to hide stuff.

I tried to distract my brother and sister by saying, 'Let's go and pack a bag you can take with you.'

I helped them find things to take with them. I got some things for myself. Everything was checked by the police.

'Here, take this. You'll need it for school,' Mum said, handing me something. 'Make sure you get all your pens and paper and your art things.'

I hesitated. What was it?

'Here you go. Jade, take it!' She was being quite forceful.

I saw that it was a pencil case but I hadn't seen it before. It certainly wasn't mine. Why did she want me to take her pencil case?

The officer was watching and she must have got suspicious because she grabbed the pencil case from Mum. She opened it and I saw there were lots of orange-capped needles and little wraps of heroin. She looked at Mum and shook her head.

Now I knew why she was so desperate for me to take it. It was her only chance to get it out of the house without being caught. She must have thought I'd know to get rid of it. She was probably right. If I had found all of that I would have thrown it in the bin.

I watched as my mother was escorted out of the house into the police van. I was shocked and dismayed by what had just happened but the overriding emotions were sadness and relief.

The social worker explained this had been a planned operation. The police had been watching the house for days and they knew they were going to have to arrest our mum. They didn't tell us exactly what she was supposed to have done wrong. We were to go to school and nursery as normal. I actually didn't mind that much. I hoped it might mean that we'd be taken into foster care and get some respite from the chaos that was life with my mother. Maybe I'd get a decent meal and be able to do something fun.

After school Shona, the social worker, was there to meet me.

'Does this mean I can go into foster care?' I asked.

'We need to see what happens about your mum in court,' she said. In the meantime we were to stay with Mum's friend. I was disappointed but anything might be better than going home with Mum.

The court granted Mum bail but she didn't return home. Neither did we. Social workers placed me with a foster carer called Sally. I'd met her before and thought she was lovely. I was delighted to be staying with her again. Shona said Jack and Ellen were going together to another carer, as much to give me some respite as she accepted I had been caring for them more than my mum.

Sally was Scottish and loved traditional dancing. Living with her, even temporarily, was a complete contrast to how things had been with Mum. She was warm and affectionate and used to cuddle me on the sofa. It was amazing to feel appreciated and not be shouted at every two seconds. She even took me on a trip to Scotland for the weekend once to meet people she knew through her dancing. They were all so upbeat and positive.

While I was having some fun at last, Mum's situation was going from bad to worse. She ended up being convicted for drug offences and serving time in Styal prison, in Cheshire. Sally took me to meet her when she was getting out. It wasn't the most touching of family reunions. Mum looked gaunter than before, haunted even, and so stick-thin. We stood outside the prison gates for a family photo. If I thought being inside might have given her time to think about what kind of mother she'd been and how she might make amends for the time we'd lost, she quickly dispelled that notion. I was still staying with Sally when, a short time later, we met with Mum. Something set her off and she slapped me viciously around my right ear. It was so hard my whole face stung and it started bleeding. My ears buzzed for hours afterwards and rang for even longer. When I got it checked out the doctor said I had a perforated eardrum. I suffered years of infections as a result.

Mum might have been out of prison but social services restricted our time with her to prearranged visits in a contact centre, normally in a community hall where they rented a room for our meeting. The social workers were there and they wouldn't leave us alone with her. Mum arrived and by the puffiness of her skin and how bloated she looked I suspected she was still on methadone. She fired questions at me about where I was staying, what I'd told people about her. Because of this, or perhaps because they suspected she might do drugs if given half a chance, she wasn't even allowed to take me or my brother or sister to the toilet on her own.

It was nice to see Jack and Ellen there. They were enjoying their temporary foster care. Ellie wanted to play and brought a toy over to me.

'Come on, Mum,' she said, pulling at my sleeve.

I looked around. Mum stood there, a stony expression on her face. The social workers didn't know where to look.

'I'm not your mum, Ellie,' I said. 'I'm your sister.'

Ellie just shrugged. It was the first time she'd called me 'Mum', but it showed how much of a role I had played in her life over the past year.

You could cut the atmosphere in the contact centre with a knife. I had never felt so embarrassed, for my mum as well, because I was scared she was going to react. I braced myself, waiting for her to kick off. She didn't usually hold back and wouldn't think twice about causing a scene in a public place and in front of social workers.

She didn't say anything, though. I think she knew. It was a damning indictment on her performance as a mother. It spoke volumes that her youngest daughter saw me, her ten-year-old sister, as her mum.

I too was speechless, for no words could express the abundance of love I had for my little sister. I felt like her protector, that I had to give more love to her because my mother showed none. I had fed her, put her to sleep and comforted her when she was upset. To hear her call me Mum meant it had not been in vain. She'd felt the love a mother should give, just not from the right person.

For some people that moment might have been a wake-up call. They might have tried cleaning up their act and working hard to rebuild the broken relationships with their children. Not our mum. All her energy went on battling her own demons and looking after her own concerns.

I remained with Sally, the foster carer, but seeing my mother only made me more desperate for the arrangement to be made permanent. It was confirmation that nothing would change. It would just be more chaos.

We carried on like this for a month, me staying with Sally, my siblings together with another foster carer. We met up for frequent visits with Mum, always under the watchful eye of social workers in a contact centre. Mum often created a scene, making comments to the social workers about taking her children off her and creating tension, so when it was time to leave, Ellen, in particular, was upset. I felt for her. How confusing this must be, to see this woman you haven't really bonded with properly claiming she wanted you back. It was confusing for all of us. I just felt embarrassed, ashamed, numb and distant from her as my mother. I saw how social workers looked at her. I knew she was making everything worse for herself. I remember thinking, why doesn't she feel embarrassed? She had absolutely no self-awareness.

Shona took me to one meeting but Mum didn't show up so she offered to take me to McDonald's to make up for it. Afterwards we still had some time to kill so she invited me back to her house to watch television until it was time to take me back to Sally's. She just wanted to give me a nice experience, but when I next met Mum I let slip what had happened. She hated the social workers anyway, and on hearing this she tried to make trouble for Shona. That led to even more animosity between them.

I prayed that the situation with Sally could be permanent. I was so happy at her house and was trying to settle at school and catch up on all the work I had missed. I longed for some stability in my life, somewhere concrete where I could make friends and feel a sense of belonging. If that couldn't be arranged, I hadn't given up hope of living with my dad. His situation continued to be complicated, however, and contact had dropped off again. Shona told me they would try to get in touch to make him aware that I was in temporary foster care.

In the back of my mind all this time was the fear that one day soon I might once again be at the mercy of my mother. She had various court hurdles to overcome and had to show that she was clean of drugs before she could get her children back.

Some of the early signs were not promising, though. After one visit, where Mum had given us each a bag of toys, there was a panic afterwards when word came through from social services that Mum had left her bottle of methadone in one of the bags. The prescription was eventually found in Ellen's bag at their foster carer's, but it was yet another indication that Mum was not ready to have us back.

And so, by October 1998, my care options were limited. Sally was unable to keep me any longer, even on an extended temporary basis. If social services did make contact with my dad again he wouldn't be able to take me, even if he wanted to, while Mum still had a chance. While she tried to sort herself out, social services worked on finding me a new temporary home.

The foster carer they settled on was seven miles away in another town. She was called Linda Black and Shona told me she was in her fifties with several grown-up children of her own. She already had two children in her care but had a large-enough house and said she could take me in as well.

Shona took me to meet her. As we pulled up outside the property I thought it looked nice. It was a terraced house that sat on the corner of a road. There were net curtains over the windows and it had a rear garden. I imagined playing there and looked around at the neighbouring houses, wondering whether there were children living there too and what they were like.

The door opened and a small lady with a big smile greeted us. She must have been only 5ft 3in tall and had a bit of a stomach. She possessed the most piercing blue eyes, jet-black hair that she wore up at the back with a short side fringe swept across her forehead and long sideburns. She wore black leather boots up to her knees that might have been imposing but for her kindly smile.

'Hello,' she said, beaming. 'You must be Jade. I've heard lots about you. All nice things of course.'

As she showed us into her home I thought, she seems nice. How bad could it be?

I had no idea.

Chapter 7

'Call me Granny,' Linda Black said, with a warm smile. 'Children in foster care can be the target for some unkind comments, so say you're staying with your grandma.'

My introduction to life at Linda's house couldn't have been better. She really did seem like a lovely old woman. She actually had a grandmotherly feel about her.

I had been a little tearful when Shona took me to my new foster home for the first time. The latest meeting with Mum had been very stressful. She spent more time kicking off about things than making use of the time she had with her children. Some things never changed, it seemed, except our living arrangements. We always seemed to be the ones to suffer. That was in my mind when we travelled to meet Linda.

When we entered the house, however, those worries quickly disappeared. Linda was happy and welcoming and immediately gave me some nice snacks to eat and showed me around her house. Downstairs there was a large kitchen, a dining room that was mostly used for storage and a living room that was big enough to have a table and chairs in it, while upstairs were three bedrooms and a bathroom. I don't think I'd ever been anywhere so big and beautiful. It was quiet because everyone else was either at work or school. Linda said her husband Terry was a builder so he left really early every morning and didn't return until the evening.

She and Terry had had six children, three girls and three boys, but only one daughter still lived with them. Her name was Lisa and she was an older teenager. I'd be sharing with her, Linda said, as she showed me upstairs and into her daughter's room. It was small, with bunk beds, and I was to take the bottom one. In the room there was a TV and a PlayStation. This was more like a holiday camp than a foster home. Linda then led me to a large room next to Lisa's at the front of the house. Inside were two sets of bunk beds, three wardrobes and three chests of drawers, one with a TV and stereo on it. There was also a wicker table and chairs. This was where the two girls she currently fostered spent most of their time. They were sisters called Arlene and Sara and had been with her for six years. Linda explained that Arlene was 12 and went to the same school as Lisa. Sara was a year older than me and attended the local high school. Linda said she'd store my clothes and what little belongings I had in one of the wardrobes.

I would still be going to the same primary school I went to at my last home. Shona said they would organise a taxi to take me there. The regular visits would continue with my mother and Jack and Ellen and they would try to arrange it so that I could see my dad again. Once Shona was happy I was settled in, she left us to it. Linda took me shopping and we had a laugh. I'd been nervous about leaving Sally's house, as I enjoyed living with her, but I soon started to think I might not miss it that much. Once again it was nice being with someone who seemed happy to have me there. Being with Linda might be the perfect alternative. After the endless chaos and drama, I longed to be part of a loving household.

When the other girls came home from school, Linda introduced us all. Arlene, the older one, was very tall, while Sara was about the same height as me, but what struck me was how skinny they were. Their clothes seemed to hang off them, they didn't say much and as they sloped upstairs I couldn't help but think there was something funny about them.

Linda's daughter Lisa, on the other hand, was a lot bubblier. It was hard to believe she was so much older as she was keen to play and excited to show me her room. I got to play on the PlayStation and watch TV before tea. It was bliss.

Terry came home in time for tea. He was big and stocky with the same piercing blue eyes as his wife. He was friendly, with a thick Mancunian accent, and he also welcomed me to the house. Both he and Linda seemed to love looking after children. Aside from the foster kids they took in, she said they also had two children from Chernobyl who came over every summer to stay. 'They're children who live in an area exposed to radiation from the nuclear disaster years ago,' Linda explained. 'Spending six weeks in England in the summer can add two years to their lives.'

Wow, I thought. This must be such a nice place to be if it has that much of an effect.

Linda made tea and I sat down with her, Terry and Lisa. Oddly, the two sisters didn't eat with us. I watched as Linda put their plates on trays at the foot of the stairs and called them one by one. They trudged down, collected them and went back upstairs.

'They have their meals in their room,' Linda said. 'They're troublesome girls. They've had difficult lives but they play up. It's best if you don't have that much to do with them.'

Fair enough, I thought. I had no idea how long I was going to be there. It didn't bother me if they didn't want to be friends.

After tea I went upstairs to get some things from the wardrobe. For some reason I was nervous about entering the room, but I went in and found the girls sitting on the floor in silence at opposite ends. They were already in their nightdresses. Their plates were on the floor beside them. It didn't look like they'd used the table and chairs. The telly wasn't on and no music was playing. Had they had a fall-out? Were they just boring? I paused for a second to see if they would say anything but they just sat there. There was something haunted about them. What was it with them? I didn't hang about to find out. I got my things and headed out, closing the door behind me. It was a bit odd. I was glad I wasn't spending the night in there.

By contrast, I played some more with Lisa and watched some TV with Linda and Terry until it was time for bed. She liked the soaps so I was happy to sit with her while she watched *Coronation Street* and *EastEnders*. Later, as I lay in my bunk that night, I thought I could get used to this house. There were worse places to be. I worked out that in the last three or four years I'd moved eleven times, and been in several women's refuges, hostels and respite homes. I didn't know how long I would be in here until it was time to go back with Mum, but I was determined to enjoy it while it lasted.

Linda's wider family came round to welcome me. They all seemed really nice, too. I got on particularly well with her daughter Rebecca and daughter-in-law Deborah, who were both in their twenties but took an interest in me and helped make me feel at home. They made a comment or two about the other girls, but not about them being badly behaved or being punished for anything. Rebecca said they always seemed to be playing in their room when they came round and Deborah said at least with them upstairs it wasn't too rowdy for Terry when he came home after a hard day on a building site. I didn't think too much of it. The girls might keep to themselves but there was no tension or a sense that they were any worse than any other children. It wasn't my concern, though. I would just concentrate on being a good girl and not giving my new foster carers any reason to think I was difficult.

For my next visit to see Mum, a taxi picked me up after school to take me to the contact centre. Mum was in a better mood than last time and told me to remember that things had been good in the past and as soon as she got herself sorted they would be good again. I just nodded. I was more concerned about Jack and Ellen and how they were coping, but they seemed to be settling in quite well with their carers.

I was enjoying life at Linda and Terry's. At the weekend, they took us all to the shops. Arlene and Sara came too but they didn't say much. They just traipsed around looking miserable. Maybe Linda was right and I should give them a wide berth. I played around with Lisa and left them to their own devices. On Saturday night I got to watch *Casualty* with Linda. Whatever the other girls got up to didn't bother me. I might not be in the house for long anyway.

Social services paid regular visits to check how I had settled in. I could genuinely tell them I was happy. They still didn't know how long we'd remain in foster care. It was now December and Shona said nothing would be decided before Christmas, so I knew we'd be spending the festivities apart. I wasn't sure what to think about that. It had been such a long time since we'd had a normal Christmas, when we went to the social club. The last two had been spent in a women's refuge. I might have been upset but in the run-up to Christmas Mum didn't show up for some of the arranged visits. On one occasion she claimed to be locked in the house. When I heard that I just thought: what's the point? A neighbour of Mum's saw me at school and said she was ill and that she could pass on any message that I wanted to see her. I told her not to bother. She knew the days when we were to see her. It made me sad to think she was still making excuses.

We did eventually see her briefly a week or so before Christmas. She had a bag of presents for us each, which was nice. It was actually good to see her. She was in a calm mood and for a moment there was a glimpse of what life could be like if we were all together. It was all too brief, though, and almost as soon as it began we had to leave to go to our respective carers.

The Bad Room

When Christmas morning came, Lisa and I got up early and went down to the living room where all the presents were waiting. As well as the gifts Mum had given me, there were parcels from Linda too. I was delighted to receive a new backpack, clothes and things for school. Arlene and Sara opened their presents in their room but came down to spend some time with the rest of us. Later in the day, Linda's children visited and we all had dinner together. It was really nice and even though I couldn't get to spend the day with my own family I felt happy to be welcomed into such a caring household.

With Linda I got to experience things I hadn't had a chance to before – things other children my age take for granted. She took me swimming, which was something I'd only done once before with Mum when she'd taken me to a local leisure centre and I nearly drowned. She'd given me armbands to wear but as usual wasn't properly supervising me. I took them off to go down a big slide and when I landed in the deep end I couldn't get back up to the surface. Someone had to rescue me. With Linda it was a lot less stressful and I found I actually enjoyed it.

I also went to the cinema for the very first time. Lisa was a member of a cinema art club, where they told children a week in advance what movie they'd be going to see so they could draw a picture on the same theme. When I went along for the first time the movie was *Free*

Willy, about a killer whale being rescued from its cruel owners. I'd heard about the cinema, obviously, but had never experienced it. I was excited to be going with Linda and Lisa. It was fun to get the popcorn and choose a drink. I sat mesmerised, as much by the adverts and trailers on the big screen as the main event. It was occasions like this that made me think it wouldn't be so bad if I ended up here on a more permanent basis.

As 1999 began that scenario looked ever more likely. At one of my first meetings with Mum since Christmas she was late, and when she arrived her eyes were like pinpricks. I knew what that meant. She said to the social worker that she hadn't been able to get her methadone prescription and had 'dabbled' in other things. She'd been in prison again, for what I didn't know. Given she still had to prove she was capable of cleaning up her act it didn't look like we would be returning home anytime soon, wherever home was. I did wonder if Mum's continued problems might make living with Dad more of a possibility, but social services were not forthcoming. Everything was up in the air. At one point it was suggested that Jack might go to live with Sally, the woman who looked after me for a while. I was still allowed to see her occasionally for tea and I thought that would be a great idea. I hoped it might mean that I could see both her and Jack. Then Shona suggested that Ellen might come to live with me at Linda's. That would have been amazing. Almost as soon as it was suggested, however, social services decided against it. There was talk that Paul might be coming out of prison soon and I wasn't sure if that had a bearing on where we were all sent.

Mum's situation got increasingly bizarre. She broke her leg in two places and turned up for our meeting in plaster. Despite this she told Jack and Ellen they'd be back with her imminently and they needed to choose which bunk bed they'd be sleeping in. At the same time this was going on I had to deal with the process of changing schools. Although I was in my final year of primary school, social services said I should move to a local school near Linda's first and then, if I was still living there come September, I would attend the same high school as Sara. As I'd missed so much schooling over the years I had to undertake additional learning hours to prepare me for an upcoming SATs test that would determine what level I went into.

It was hard work but I'd enjoyed being back at school and did well enough in the test to get a good placing. As I prepared to start my new primary school in spring that year, Linda reiterated the advice she'd given me initially: 'Just tell people I'm your granny. Kids can pick on foster children.'

She also told me not to be seen walking out to school with Sara. Even though my primary school was five minutes from the house and she had to walk a further 15 minutes to the high school, Linda said: 'You do not want to be associated with her. People round here know she's in care. You'll get off on completely the wrong foot.'

In my nice new uniform I made sure I left at a different time to Sara, who made the walk to school alone. I was apprehensive about starting yet another new school. It was bad enough making yet another transition from a different town but even worse that I wasn't at home and was living in foster care. I did as Linda said and told people I'd recently moved into the area and was living with my granny. Despite my reticence, the girls I met were nice and keen to be friends. They would soon be going to the same high school as me if I stayed on at Linda's. Instinctively, I kept my guard up to some extent, but it was a relief to meet children on my wavelength. Just as it had been with Linda, my first impression was that I might once more enjoy life at school.

I should have known, though, that just when I was beginning to think things might be settling down into something resembling a routine, it would all kick off. I don't know what she had done this time but Mum was back in prison. I did feel sorry for her, but I also felt sad about my own situation. It was bad enough trying to hide the fact I was in foster care but I was worried what the reaction would be if my new friends found out my mum was in prison. She wanted to see me so Shona picked me up from school one day and we travelled to

Styal Prison for a visit. I clung tightly to Shona's hand as we went in. I might have had more experience of jails than a child my age ought to, but I still found them unnerving places to enter. It didn't help that a present I'd got for her was confiscated as we went through security.

Mum's wing wasn't quite as foreboding as some I'd been in, and when I saw her I gave her a big hug. She led us through to a family room where there was a basketball and net. I immediately wanted to play but Mum wanted to speak to me first. There was obviously something going on between her and the social worker.

'She doesn't know, does she?' Mum asked Shona.

'No, we haven't told her. We felt it was up to you?'

What could it be? What did she have to tell me?

'I'm going to have another baby,' Mum said, smiling awkwardly.

'Get lost,' I said. 'You're having me on.'

'It's true, sweetheart,' Mum said.

I looked at Shona. She just nodded.

'Oh my God,' I said.

I was aware she might have been seeing someone new but I hadn't given it much thought. I didn't know what this meant. She could barely look after herself, let alone her existing three children and now she was expecting another baby.

Mum said she was testing negative for drugs and would be out of prison soon.

'Where would you like to live?' she said, meaning that we'd be together again.

I had no idea. I thought of my dad and how I hadn't seen him for a long time.

Then she dropped another bombshell. 'Paul is still in prison but I got a letter from him saying it's time you went in to see him.'

I said nothing. When I thought of Paul all that came back were thoughts of fear and pain. I did not want to see him.

By the time Shona took me back to Linda's I was emotionally exhausted. I dozed off in the car, my head spinning with thoughts of yet more turmoil. The prospect of going back to live with Mum had never felt more real – and troubling. When I considered which option presented a calmer, more settled future – going back to Mum or staying with Linda – I felt sure it was my foster carer. She appeared to be everything Mum wasn't – reliable, affectionate and caring. As I was about to find out, however, appearances can be deceptive.

Chapter 8

It came out of nothing. Or so I thought. Maybe if I had been living there for longer I might have been able to spot the signs that it was about to kick off.

Lisa and Arlene came home from school as normal and I looked forward to my usual games session on the PlayStation.

'Mum!' Lisa shouted, before she did anything else. 'I saw Arlene playing with Millie today.'

Arlene shot upstairs and, without a word, Linda hared up after her. I'd never seen her move so fast. They both crashed into the bedroom and the door slammed shut behind them. I could hear Linda from the bottom of the stairs, not every word but enough to get the gist.

'What have I ... playing ... that girl? I've told you ... slag!'

'That's my best friend!' I heard Arlene reply. 'Don't be calling her names.'

Lisa was listening too, almost giggling with every outburst but with a mock look of shock on her face, as if to say, 'Oh my, have I said something wrong?'

I suspected this wasn't the first time she'd told tales from school. I had no idea who this Millie was but I guessed she was a bad influence in Linda's eyes.

They were still shouting, until I heard Arlene scream, 'Leave me alone!'

Then there was the unmistakable sound of a smack. Then another. There was a scuffle and then the door swung open and slammed before Linda stormed downstairs. Lisa and I ducked into the kitchen.

'I've told her so many times not to mix with that Millie. That girl's trouble. Well done for telling me.'

She treated Lisa to some sweets and by now had completely calmed down. I was surprised at her reaction but I thought the Millie girl must really be a piece of work to merit that response.

'What is it with those two?' I asked Linda.

'They're just very naughty. They need to be disciplined, otherwise they run riot. It's for their own good. You just keep away from them and don't have anything to do with them. They're brats. You can't trust them.'

Lisa giggled, still revelling in her role in all of this.

Linda cooked dinner but didn't leave out two plates of what Lisa and I were having for Arlene and Sara. Instead, two plates with a meagre ham sandwich on each were laid out. She called them and they trudged down, sighed when they saw it and headed back upstairs with their plates.

Maybe it's because of the way I was raised, with Mum not really treating me like a child, or perhaps it's due to always being around adults as a youngster but I have always had a tendency to pay closer attention to the behaviour of grown-ups than most children my age. After our meal was cleared up I watched as Linda climbed the stairs slowly and hovered around at the top on the landing. It was like she was waiting on something. Suddenly she burst into the room. 'Who was talking? I said, "No talking." Neither of you will be getting any tea at all tomorrow at this rate.'

'No one was talking,' I heard Sara say. I certainly hadn't heard anything.

'Are you saying I imagined it? Tell me which one of you was talking.'

There was a bit of backchat. I couldn't hear what was said. I only heard Linda's response. A loud whack.

'Ow!'

I wasn't sure if that was Arlene or Sara.

Now I heard Arlene's voice. 'My own mum never used to hit me, so why can you?'

'Don't you speak to me like that!' There was another whack.

'Go straight to bed! Now!'

After what sounded like a bit of a scuffle, Linda came out of the room and closed the door. I nipped back into the kitchen so she wouldn't catch me looking. I didn't hear her come down the stairs so I peeked round the door and nearly got a fright. She was standing on the stairs, just a few steps down. She was still looking up at the door so she hadn't seen me. There was silence from the room but she was clearly listening out for something. She must have heard it for she jumped back up the last remaining steps and threw open the door again. 'I said silence! I warned you. No tea tomorrow.'

I heard one of the girls complain. 'But we weren't making any noise.'

Linda left the room and closed the door once more. She came downstairs but sat at the dining room table, smoking, listening for sounds of any noise. Terry was in the same room as her, watching television, seemingly oblivious to what was going on upstairs. Lisa and I got ready for bed, but just as we were about to climb into our bunks I heard Linda race up the stairs again. It was amazing how fast she could move for someone her size.

'Someone has been up to go to the toilet. Who was it?'

I could hear the girls protest but it was no good. Linda was on the warpath and determined to punish them.

In the morning I didn't think much more about the events of the previous night. I went to school, came home and everything seemed normal. I played with

The Bad Room

Lisa and the girls were in their room as usual. It was only at teatime when I saw that no plates at all were left out for Arlene and Sara that I remembered. They were to go without their tea tonight.

'Was your mum serious?' I said to Lisa, discreetly. 'Are they not getting anything to eat?'

Lisa just shrugged. Sure enough, though, while we ate, Linda left nothing out for the sisters. They were not called down. They had been in their room since they came home from school. I carried on as normal and played with Lisa and didn't really think much more about it. They had misbehaved and disobeyed Linda and this was their punishment. It wasn't anything to do with me.

It was late spring and the evenings were getting lighter. The sun was still streaming in through the windows when I needed to go into the girls' room to get something from the wardrobe. The room was so quiet I pushed the door gently. The latch didn't work on the door but it jammed a bit and you had to give it a push to open. I did so. There was a bit of a squeaking noise when I stepped inside. You wouldn't have thought there was anyone in the room because it was so still and quiet, so I got a fright when the two figures on the floor turned with a start to look at me. The curtains were drawn so the room was darker than the rest of the house, although shafts of light seeped through the sides and the top of the drapes. The girls looked like ghostly figures, sitting there, at opposite ends of the room, already in their nighties. Sara hugged her knees tight to her chest, her nightdress pulled over her legs. There was a horrible smell, a musty mix of stale urine and body odour. Outside I could hear the excited chatter of other children playing elsewhere in the street. That was something none of us were allowed to do, go out and play. We were all to stay in the house after school, but nothing was as bad as this. I looked around. All they had to play with was a box of Lego. There were a couple of notepads and pens too for amusement. And that was it. The TV remained unplugged. The stereo looked like it was there for show only.

They both looked relieved to see it was just me. Maybe they expected it was Linda. But once they got over their initial shock they shot me a look of contempt. I got my things from the wardrobe and headed back to the door. I didn't want to hang around in there longer than was necessary. It was so gloomy and grim.

'That was us for the first year,' Sara said quietly.

The suddenness of her words gave me a fright but I quickly composed myself. 'What?'

'That's how it was for us when we first moved here.'

'What are you on about?'

'It was all nice and friendly,' Arlene said, scowling. 'Nice food, treats, getting to play games, staying up watching TV.'

'So?' I said.

'Then it changes,' Sara said. 'You get shouted at, hit, punished, for every little thing. Even when you do nothing wrong.'

I laughed. It was obvious they were just trying to freak me out or make me miserable, because they'd been in the wrong. I remembered what Linda said about them being naughty. You couldn't trust them, she'd said. Was this what she meant? Were they twisting things to make them look hard done by? It did seem harsh not to get any dinner but they had done something to annoy Linda. Clearly they should have learned not to get in her bad books. I shrugged and moved closer to the door. I didn't want to linger in there. There was such a bad vibe.

'Mark my words,' Sara said. She wasn't even looking at me now. Her head was bowed, her eyes fixed on a point on the floor.

'Whatever,' I said, trying not to sound like I was freaked out. 'I might not be here for much longer anyway. I'm probably going back to my mum.'

Arlene shrugged. 'That's what we thought.'

'Yeah, but my case is different. I'll be finding out soon.'

Arlene stared at me, her eyes like pools of black in the half-light. 'You'll see.'

I thought about saying something back but was overcome with an urge to just get out of there. It was so spooky I half feared the door would shut and I'd be trapped in there with them.

The Bad Room

I got out of the room, closed the door and went through to the other bedroom, relieved to be back out in the daylight. I rejoined Lisa and we played some more before it was time to go to bed. I didn't see the girls again that night, not even at shower time when we got ready for bed. There was none of the same drama of the night before. Linda was in and out of their room but I never heard a peep all evening.

That night, as I lay awake in bed, I was relieved to be where I was, in a room with Linda's daughter and not in with them. I didn't know what the story was with those girls, nor did I know whether I'd be here long enough to find out, but I knew one thing – there was a weird vibe in that room. It was a bad room. I did not want to be stuck in there.

Chapter 9

I had a feeling something bad was going to happen the moment Linda sat me down and said she wanted to tell me something. I had just come home from school and immediately started worrying that I had done something wrong.

She said she had a stomach ulcer and bowel problems and was going to be going into hospital in the next few days for an operation. Before then and when she came out she wanted to be in Lisa's room so Terry wouldn't be disturbed.

'I need to move you out of Lisa's room,' she said.

It wasn't what I was expecting, but I began to panic. No, please. This couldn't be.

'I'm going to move you in with Arlene and Sara.'

'No,' I pleaded, feeling the tears well up. 'Not in there – with them. I don't want to go in that room.'

'I need your bed, I need to move out of my room temporarily. It will only be for a short time.'

Certainly she hadn't looked well for a while and wasn't jumping up and down the stairs like she used up. I could see she was ill. But this was still a nightmare. It was everything I didn't want to happen. All I could think of was sitting there, on the floor, hour after hour, doing nothing. In there with those two girls who no doubt hated me.

'Do I have to?' I kept saying.

'I'm not well, Jade. I can't sleep. I'm keeping Terry awake at night and it's not fair on him. He needs his rest. He gets up at 5.30 every morning.'

She was probably telling me the truth. All I heard was that I was going in there. Into the 'Bad Room'.

I heard what she was saying but I still felt like I was being punished.

'Please don't put me in there. I don't want to go in there with those two. They don't like me. You said you stay away from them. I can go somewhere else.'

'Don't be silly. There are beds in there. It makes sense. Those two are not too bad as long as they behave themselves.'

'But I won't be able to come downstairs. I'll have to stay in there. Please, no.'

'You can still come downstairs,' Linda said. 'It won't be that bad. It's only for a short time. Then you can go back in with Lisa.'

I couldn't argue my case anymore. She'd made up her mind. I felt really uneasy about it. I watched as she hobbled up the stairs and made a bed up for me. I was to sleep in the bottom bunk, below Sara.

'We told you,' Sara said when Linda finished and went back downstairs.

'It's not like that,' I said. 'It's only for a short time, until she gets better. You'll see.'

She exchanged a look with Arlene, one that said, 'Yeah, right.'

'Can I put the telly on in the room?' I asked Linda.

'No, that television is not to be put on. Those two aren't allowed to watch TV. If you want to watch something you need to ask Lisa if you can watch it on hers.'

'What about the stereo? Can I listen to music?'

'No, they aren't allowed that either.'

I didn't see the point of having them in the room. They might as well have been ornaments. I didn't argue though. At least I could still watch TV. And Linda was true to her word; I didn't have to eat my tea in the room with the girls, I could still hang out with Lisa in her room and I was also still able to watch television downstairs with Terry and her.

'See,' I said, when I finally went to bed, after they'd been stuck in the room for ages. 'You're wrong. It's not the same.'

They just shrugged. I didn't care. I resolved to spend as little time in that room as possible. I got nervous every time Linda closed the door, as though one time it would be slammed shut and we'd never get out.

I needn't have worried, however, because when Linda went into hospital for her operation it was like we all had a bit of a holiday. Terry was off work and when he was around the whole atmosphere was more relaxed. He let us come and go as we pleased. We got to play outside after school and the girls were allowed out of their room. As long as we helped with the meals and tidied up, Terry was happy. It was the first time all four of us girls actually had some fun together. I saw a side to Arlene and Sara I hadn't seen before. They didn't seem that bad actually.

When Linda came home she looked very poorly. It seemed to take all of her energy to get to the sofa where she could lie and watch TV. We were still a bit on 'Terry mode' and were used to getting our own way. What made it worse was that I'd had my first sex education class at school that day and was in a giggly mood, desperate to share with the other girls the excruciating videos I'd watched. Arlene and Sara had already experienced the same videos so at night we were upstairs laughing at how embarrassing we found it. Even after we were supposed to be asleep the two sisters kept remembering something and getting a fit of the giggles. Before Linda went into hospital they would never have carried on like this. It was as though not having her around had given them a new lease of life. And with me in their room they had a bit of an audience. We were all sitting up in bed. I'd lost track of the time but it was probably quite late. I wasn't find-ing the sex stuff as funny anymore and was thinking we should call it a night. I told them to be quiet but they ignored me.

'It's not like she's going to run upstairs, is she?' Arlene said.

Just as she said it the door swung open and there was Linda, raised from her sick bed, looking furious.

We all jumped out of our skins.

'For once would you all just do as you are told?'

She hobbled into the room clutching her stomach.

'What time do you call this? Why are you not asleep?'

'Sorry, we were just chatting,' I said, looking to the others to back me up. They sat in silence.

'I expected better from you, Jade,' she said, lurching menacingly in the direction of my bunk.

'What? It wasn't just me. It was them too.'

Just as I leaned out to look up to Sara for some support Linda swung out and slapped me across the back of my head. It hurt but I was more taken aback by the shock of being hit.

'Now get to bed – and be quiet!'

She hobbled out of the room and closed the door behind her. I couldn't believe she had hit me, and if she was going to hit anyone at all, why just me and not the others too? Did she seriously believe I was the one at fault?

I buried my head in my pillow, hurt and confused. I thought she liked me and treated me differently. In the darkness I could hear the girls whispering. I imagined the smug looks on their faces. Were they right? Was this how it was going to be for me now?

As for Arlene and Sara, they were happy to sit there and keep quiet and let me take the blame.

Half term was approaching and I was excited to be seeing my brother and sister. All three of us went into prison to visit Mum, who was still serving her sentence. I told Mum Linda had hit me. She asked Shona, the social worker who'd accompanied us, if she knew about it. She said no. I hadn't told her yet.

'Do you want me to investigate further?' Shona said.

'Do you?' Mum asked me.

Suddenly I had second thoughts. I didn't want a big inquiry. It might make things worse.

'Just leave it,' I said. 'It wasn't a big deal.'

'Are you sure?' Mum said. 'Foster carers shouldn't be hitting children, should they?'

'No, they shouldn't,' Shona said.

'It's fine, just leave it.' I was trying to get into Linda's good books again. There had been no incidents since that night. I didn't want to give her a reason to pick on me.

'Only if you're sure, Jade,' Shona said.

I thought we were leaving it at that but a few days later Shona arrived at the house with a colleague, a family placement officer called Brenda. They said Mum's lawyer had written to social services requesting they investigate it. They asked Linda if she had smacked me across the head.

'Yes,' Linda said. She went on to tell how she'd been in hospital for a major operation and came home to find us all acting loudly and naughtily. We had been making a racket upstairs and she had been unable to get upstairs to tell us to quieten down because of her post-operative state, which meant she'd be sleeping on the sofa. She painted quite a picture. I wondered if she was talking about the same night. It was past 11.30 p.m. and we were still making a racket in the bedroom, jumping up and down and making disgusting 'sexy talk' and noises. I couldn't believe what she was saying.

Eventually, she had no option, she said, but to haul herself off the sofa, stagger up the stairs, enter the room and tell us off. She said she cuffed me around the back of the head to make her point as I was being cheeky and answering back.

Shona and Brenda asked Linda to demonstrate what she did. She showed the open-handed slap she'd dished out, only this time it looked like a gentle brush, as opposed to the whack I'd received.

The social workers reminded Linda about the council's 'no smacking' policy.

'I'm well aware of that and usually follow it to the

letter,' Linda said, 'but they were playing up and it was too much in my state of health.'

Shona did speak to me on my own afterwards but by now I just wanted to forget the whole incident. I hated it being picked over and there was no way Linda was going to admit she'd overreacted. Shona said that because I hadn't suffered any injuries and because I'd said previously I was happy at Linda's and hadn't reported any other cases of mistreatment she was not going to consider it physical abuse. They'd put it down to an isolated incident.

Shona said that if anything like that happened again I should tell someone, but I didn't like how the whole episode had played out. Maybe I should have spoken out more but it was embarrassing hearing adults going on about the 'sexy talk' and us mucking about.

Mum got out of prison a week later but it was still unclear what was going to happen to us all. She was pregnant, still on methadone and as erratic as ever. I was due to see her before my eleventh birthday but she cancelled, claiming she wasn't feeling well. Linda, instead, threw a little party for me at the house, which I hoped was a sign I was back in favour again.

She was still recuperating and sleeping in Lisa's room but quickly got back to her old ways with her treatment of Arlene and Sara. I was relieved to find that even after the episode with the social workers she still allowed me to eat downstairs. The sisters, however, continued to be confined to their room.

Since we'd got into trouble relations were frosty between us. I didn't trust them and spent as little time as possible in the room. This seemed to please Linda, who continued to give them a hard time.

Although Arlene appeared perfectly able, she wasn't allowed to go to any parties or after-school activities. This used to drive her mad and she'd kick off about always being left out.

Then Lisa would come home and tell her mum she saw Arlene talking to boys at school. Linda would immediately take this up with Arlene, calling her a slag and punishing her by sending her to bed early or making her go without her tea.

Lisa also told on Arlene any time she saw her speaking to her friend Millie, which was a lot. That led to yet another argument and then Linda would punish both of them for talking when they shouldn't be or making even the tiniest of noises. Sara was forever coughing and sniffing. She got every bug that was going around. Any time she sniffed too loudly or had a coughing fit, Linda was up there screaming at her. She thought they were deliberately taking the mickey out of her.

After one blazing row with them, Linda claimed to know things about the girls that would explain why she had to be so hard on them. When I asked what, she said things that were so mean and inappropriate I couldn't believe they were true. I was shocked she would even say such things to me. It made me wonder what she was saying to them in return.

Now that I was sharing a room with them at night I could see how miserable their lives were. Simple pleasures – like being able to eat when you want, have treats, watch some TV – things that I was allowed to do, were forbidden for them.

On a good day they just had their three meals a day. They regularly went without their dinner, however, or had to go to bed straight from school without a bath or shower. Sometimes Linda just made them sit on the floor, at opposite ends of the room, with their backs to each other, not speaking or doing anything. She checked on them every few minutes to make sure they were still in the same positions.

'It's to give them time to think about how badly behaved they've been,' Linda said.

I felt sorry for them but part of me thought rather them than me. By contrast I felt quite spoiled. I went downstairs when I wanted, ate with the family and watched television or played on Lisa's PlayStation. Social services were constantly monitoring my situation and making sure I was happy.

And I was.

Even for the other girls there were moments of genuine fun. When Terry had time off work he and Linda took all four of us girls to a holiday park an hour's drive away. We stayed in a caravan and it was brilliant. We went swimming during the day and at night we watched the entertainment. Linda entered Lisa, Sara and me into a talent competition. The organisers dressed me in a black curly wig and I pretended to be Cher singing her recent big hit 'Believe'. I won the contest and the prize was another holiday for us all for the camp's closing party in November.

For a few weeks in the summer the two girls from Chernobyl visited. To accommodate them, Linda moved back into her room and moved Lisa in there too, giving the Ukrainians the bunk beds. Their English wasn't very good and they kept themselves to themselves, only really mixing with us at the weekend when we all went shopping. They were a year or two older than me but looked a lot more mature, with heavy make-up and winged eyeliner. Although they were meant to be suffering from the effects of radiation from the fallout from the Chernobyl nuclear power station disaster in 1986, you would never have known they were poorly. But, as Linda said, spending time in the UK added two years to their life expectancy, and while they stayed any tensions or arguments in the house ceased.

So as we approached the end of the school summer holidays in 1999 I was in a good place. I felt settled at school, was getting to grips with the subjects and for the first time had made genuine friends.

What I didn't realise was that behind the scenes moves were taking place to decide my future. The first I learned about it was when Shona came to the house for what I thought was one of her regular visits.

'I have some news for you,' she said. 'It concerns your mum, now she's out of prison and expecting another baby. She plans to move to another part of England, to a big city, with her new partner.'

I stared at her blankly, trying to understand the implications.

'Do you want to move there with her?'

'Does she want me to?'

'She says she does but there are concerns about her ability to properly care for you and Jack and Ellen.'

Just a few months earlier it felt like I might be moving back with Mum, but since then she'd been back in prison, back on drugs, I'd received the bombshell news about her baby and everything had been thrown up in the air again. I missed my brother and sister so much but thinking about living with Mum again brought back memories of the chaos. Playing the role of mother to them both had been exhausting. Would it be like that all over again? In addition, the thought of moving to a new city and having to go through the process of starting a new school, making friends all over again, was too much. I had the daunting prospect of starting a new high school but at least I'd met people who were going there. No one knew I was in care. I was a bit apprehensive about making the step up, but doing it in a completely new environment seemed a worse prospect.

'No,' I said. 'I do not want to move to a new city.'

'Do you want to stay here?' Shona asked.

I asked what my options were. Shona said she had made contact with my dad again but his situation had not changed. He was concerned to learn I was in foster care but his hands were tied. He had his partner to consider and there was the fact that Mum was still against me living with him, even if she was unable to look after me. I asked if I could see him again. She said she would look into arranging that.

It felt like an easy decision to make. Linda wasn't perfect but on the whole she had been kind to me, she didn't treat me like the other girls in her care and I enjoyed our holidays and playing with Lisa.

'Will I still get to see Jack and Ellen and have contact with my mum and dad?' I asked.

'Yes. Perhaps not as frequently as before, but you will still have contact.'

Shona made good on her promise, setting up a meeting with my dad. It was the first time I'd seen him in years. When we met in a McDonald's he gave me a big hug and I realised how much I had missed him. We spent a bit of time catching up, him telling me how his side of the family were and me filling him in on life at Linda's and what Mum was like.

He apologised to me for losing touch but said it had been almost impossible to keep track of us during our many moves. He had tried to help our situation when he could by giving us a food hamper and giving me toys and bikes but he knew Paul stole all the bikes he gave me and suspected Mum sold some of the other presents he handed over.

With Shona's approval, we made plans to meet every week on a Monday after that. I came away overjoyed that we'd made contact again but at the back of my mind I worried what Mum's reaction would be.

When I next saw Dad it was two weeks later, due to a bank holiday. He took me shopping and bought me lots of stationery and a pair of trainers for starting high school. As a belated birthday present he also gave me a radio with headphones that looked like a portable CD Walkman but was actually a secret diary with a screen inside to write entries on. When we parted he vowed to see me in a week's time. It was exciting to have him back in my life after all this time.

When I got home I showed Linda and Lisa my radio. I loved it. I'd missed listening to music so much. It had been a big part of my life with Mum, before drugs took her over, and I was thrilled to hear the latest tunes and reconnect with songs I'd not heard for a couple of years. It was my most prized possession and every chance I got I took off to a quiet spot of the house with my headphones in, lost in the music.

Later that week I went to meet Mum with Jack and Ellen at a local contact centre. She was very late and arrived looking excitable and scatty. It looked like she was under the influence of something. I said I'd seen Dad and told her about the gifts he'd bought me.

She made a comment like, 'Well, he would do that, wouldn't he?'

'It was for my birthday,' I said.

Her tone suddenly softened. 'Did you tell him about me? Did you tell him I was okay and that I'm getting better? Everyone deserves a second chance.'

I said I'd try to pass that on.

I didn't get the chance though. When I was due to meet Dad the following week he didn't show up and Shona couldn't reach him. I was disappointed, but seeing him again had given me a real boost ahead of starting high school. Making that step up to secondary school is a big moment for any child but my mind was in turmoil with Mum's situation. At least Linda presented some form of stability and I liked the friends I'd made since moving to this town. No one at school knew I was in foster care and I was keen to keep it that way. The last thing I wanted was people gossiping about me. I could only imagine what type of comments there would be if they found out my mum had been in prison and was a drug addict.

Linda was supportive on that front and even though

Sara and I were now at the same school she reiterated that I should have nothing to do with her.

'Don't leave the house together and don't be seen talking to her. She can walk to school and you can take the bus, until you get settled.'

That suited me fine. I wanted to carve out my own identity without people judging me.

It would have been nice to be able to tell my parents how I found high school but I couldn't. Since those two meetings with Dad, social services said they'd been unable to reach him. I was confused and upset. Did he not want to see me? I hoped the matter could be resolved and I lived in hope that our meetings would resume soon.

At the same time Mum's contact visits were very erratic. When she did appear she was animated and acting bizarre but often the meetings were cancelled, invariably at short notice. I felt like she had given up; that she had a new relationship and was moving away and didn't want us in her life any more.

In December Shona told me Mum had been admitted to hospital and had given birth to a little girl. She named her Abbie. I wouldn't get to see her though. Social services took her into care almost immediately.

That same month Shona told me a court had made me the subject of something known as a section 34:4 order, which meant that I was now in the permanent care of Linda Black. The implications of what she said didn't really sink in. I had known it was coming, and apart from wanting the contact with my dad to resume again I didn't want anything else to change.

Little did I know, though, that the issuing of that court order would change everything. Nothing would ever be the same again – as I was about to find out to my cost.

Chapter 10

'Jade?' Linda said, as I came through the door. We were nearing the end of term when we'd break up for Christmas. Nothing in the tone of her voice gave a hint of what was about to happen next.

'Yes?' I called through to the living room.

'Can you just go upstairs to your room and stay in there?'

If I'd had any inkling of what this meant I might have protested, fought my corner, done anything to stop it happening. I just thought she might be busy, or not feeling well and wanted us out of her hair. I felt sure she would soon call me down for my tea and later I'd be able to watch *Coronation Street* and *EastEnders* with her and Terry or play with Lisa. I had the radio my dad gave me so I lay on my bed, put my headphones in and listened to music. Arlene and Sara came home and were a bit surprised to see me sitting in the room.

There was still a lot of distrust between us. They didn't like the fact that I got special privileges, while I didn't like it when they caused noise and then joined forces to try to get me into trouble.

I was still upstairs when the call came for Sara to get her dinner plate. I jumped up and ran down while Sara sloped after me. I stopped at the foot of the stairs. There were three trays lying there. There was no cooked food, just three sandwiches with what looked like ham in them, plus a cup of water on each.

I jumped past them and went into the kitchen, expecting to see my real dinner sitting there.

'Eat your dinner in your room, Jade,' Linda said, her face expressionless.

'Have I done something wrong?'

Lisa was there but she wasn't making eye contact.

'Eat your dinner upstairs, Jade, with the other girls.' Linda wasn't even looking at me now.

Two plates remained at the foot of the stairs. Sara was halfway up, holding hers, while Arlene waited at the top for her call. It was confirmation that this wasn't a mistake and I was being treated the same as them. I trudged back up after her and took my plate into the room.

'Told you,' Arlene said, as Linda called her and she prepared to pass me.

'What?'

'That it would happen to you. That's how it was for us. Nicey nicey for a few months and then she turns.'

'Shut up!' I said. I didn't want to believe that she was right.

When Arlene returned to our room they both sat on the floor, cross-legged, their plates on their knees. I pulled a chair out at the table.

'You're not allowed to sit there,' Arlene said.

'Why not? It's what it's there for. It's a table and chairs.'

'You'll see,' Sara said.

I hated it when they talked like that, like they knew everything. It was bad enough that I had to eat in my room but why were we not allowed to use the table? It didn't make any sense. I sat down and looked at the sandwich. Two pieces of dry bread with a slice of wafer-thin ham. My stomach groaned as though even it could tell already that wasn't going to fill me up.

Suddenly the door swung open.

'A bit too much talking going on in here.' It was Linda, hands on hips, tapping one of her knee-length-boot-clad feet on the floor. 'Who was it?'

'Jade.' They both spoke as one.

'Was not!'

'Jade, now you're in this room you need to learn to keep it quiet. I don't want to hear any noise from this room when you're in here. Do you understand? And who said you could sit at the table?'

'Where else are we supposed to sit?'

'The floor. Like those two. I don't want you making a mess of my good table. And don't answer back. For that you can go straight to bed as soon as you've finished that.'

'But it's only six o'clock,' I said.

'Well, then, you shouldn't be cheeky.'

I could swear Arlene and Sara were stifling giggles. They must love this, I thought. As Linda left the room and closed the door I realised I had no option but to eat my tea and do as she said. I finished my plate, took it back downstairs and put my nightie on. It was the same one I'd had when I first moved to the house and it was starting to get small for me. I would need to speak to her about getting a new one.

I lay in bed for a bit but when the others were having their showers I got up to use the bathroom. Linda was there with Lisa. Even though she was 19 years old her mother oversaw every aspect of her life, even showering.

'Where do you think you're going?' Linda said.

'To the toilet.'

'No you're not. I told you to go straight to bed.'

'But I need to go. I'll wet the bed otherwise.'

'That's your problem. Maybe you won't be so cheeky. And it's your fault for having too much to drink earlier.'

What was she on about? I couldn't believe she wasn't letting me use the toilet. I'd heard her use similar threats with the other two girls but I always assumed they got to go. Then I remembered the times the room smelt of stale urine.

'Please,' I said. 'Can I just go? I'll be quick and I'll be better tomorrow.'

'Go to bed!' Linda screamed.

I did as I was told but within an hour of us all going to bed I really was bursting. I got up and went to the door.

'What are you doing?' Arlene's voice sounded in the darkness.

'Going to the toilet.'

'I wouldn't do that.'

'Why?'

'You'll see. She'll go mental.'

'Then I'll be careful. She won't catch me.'

'She will,' Sara whispered. 'She always does.'

I tried to open the door slowly. It was stuck, like it had been jammed in. I'd never really studied the door before. I knew the latch didn't work but didn't really know how it stayed shut.

'You're going to get into so much trouble,' Arlene whispered.

I gave the door a tug. It opened with that squeak I'd heard before. I caught my breath. It was a bit loud but there wasn't any movement outside the room so I scolded myself for being so jittery. This was nonsense. You couldn't stop someone from going to the bathroom. Nevertheless I peered outside and checked along the landing. There was no one there. Lisa would be in bed and Linda and Terry must be downstairs watching TV. I could hear the noise from the telly in the living room. I walked slowly to the bathroom. I'd never noticed how squeaky the floorboards were. It's only when you're trying to be quiet that you start spotting how loud things are. I got to the bathroom and finally relieved myself. It felt good. I pulled the flush, washed my hands and went back along to the room. The door was as I left it. I snuck inside and closed the door quietly behind me, pushing it over to see if it would stick.

'See,' I said, turning round into the darkness. 'That wasn't so …'

I nearly jumped out of my skin.

Someone was standing right in front of me. It was Linda!

'Think you can defy me, do you? Think you're better than everyone?'

'No,' I said, not knowing whether to dive into bed or stand there.

The answer came quick enough.

'Get …' Slap!

'Into …' Slap!

'Bed.'

I ducked past her but felt a blow with each word. I dived under the covers and pulled them over my head. She whacked me over the covers for good measure.

'Don't you ever defy me again!' she yelled. 'Understood?'

'Yes. Sorry,' I said meekly, heart thumping.

She left the room, at least I think she did. I remained under the covers, not wanting to poke my head out in case she was still there waiting to hit me again. What had happened? Was it something I'd done, or said? Why was she being so mean?

'We told you,' one of the girls whispered.

I didn't answer. I just stayed tucked tightly under the covers trying to make sense of the day's events. I wasn't like them. Linda had said so. She must just be in a bad mood. It would all be better in the morning.

When I got up I got dressed and made sure I was first down as usual for breakfast. Linda had her routine. She left out cereal for us, lined up with four bowls, next to our packed lunch for the day that usually comprised a sandwich, a biscuit, a tangerine and a carton of pop in a bag. She left these on the worktop. This morning there were only three bowls and three bags. I knew as soon as I saw them what it meant. I'd seen it often enough with Arlene and Sara; get into a fight with Linda at night, there would be no food for you the following day. Surely not, though. All I'd done was go to the toilet.

I was standing there staring at the worktop when Lisa, Arlene and Sara came in. They grabbed their bowls and started helping themselves to cereal.

'Have you seen your mum?' I said to Lisa.

She shrugged.

'Don't question it,' Arlene said, tucking into her cereal. 'Unless you want to miss your tea too.'

'Don't help her,' Sara said. 'No one told us what to do.'

Arlene sighed. 'Whatever. I'm sure she'll soon work it out.'

'I'm not like you two,' I said, trying to sound defiant. Maybe I was just trying to convince myself.

I went to find Linda. This might have just been a mistake. Or a test, to scare me after she'd had to tell me off. That was it. I'd speak to her and it would all be sorted. I'd be back down watching the soaps that night as though nothing happened.

'Excuse me, Linda, there were only three bowls laid out in the kitchen and three lunches.'

'I left out breakfast and lunch for those who deserve it.'

'But that means I won't have anything to eat.' My stomach was already starting to rumble.

'Well, you can think about how you've behaved while you're at school and if you want to be treated the same as everyone else then you need to respect the rules. Terry has to be up early every morning, as you well know, and we can't have you lot getting up all night to go to the toilet, making a racket.'

'But …'

'Are you wanting to go without your dinner as well? Because you're going the right way about it.'

'No. Sorry.'

Head bowed, I sloped out of the room.

'Oh, and Jade?'

I turned.

'Just to let you know there's no money for your bus fare anymore so you will have to walk to school like Sara. But I still don't want you speaking to her. You'll be in even more trouble if you do.'

Not wanting to be punished further, I just nodded, got my things and left for school. Turning back I saw Linda standing in the window watching me. From her front window she could see down to a pedestrian crossing. Sara left around the same time but she walked on the other side of the road to me. I imagined Sara loved this, seeing me now having to walk like her.

All day at school I was starving. Luckily one of my friends, Leanne, took pity on me and gave me a little bit of her lunch but I had hunger pangs all day. It didn't help that when I bumped into Sara she still looked like she was enjoying my fall from grace.

At school we were supposed to wear the uniform a certain way. That meant our knee socks were to be pulled all the way up. A lot of girls thought it cooler to roll them down to their ankles. When Sara had left the house she'd had them pulled up but by the time she got to school she'd rolled them down. I wanted to get back into Linda's good books and be her favourite again. This, I thought, was something she might like to hear.

I got home before Sara and told Linda what I'd seen.

'That is very interesting. Thank you for telling me that.'

I was pleased, thinking it might just be enough to win her over. I looked forward to having a shot on Lisa's PlayStation.

'Now go to your room and let me deal with it.'

I was about to complain when I thought better of it. I was so hungry I desperately didn't want to miss out on my tea.

Listening for the sound of Sara coming home I was disappointed when there didn't seem to be any confrontation. I heard her come upstairs and when she entered the room her socks were pulled up again. We exchanged tight smiles. I lay on the bed listening to my radio, feeling a twinge of embarrassment that I'd told on her and she'd managed to avoid any grief from Linda.

Just then the door swung open and there stood our foster carer, eyes wild, hands on her hips.

'So, Sara, what is this I hear about you looking like a scrubber at school?'

'What?' Sara's voice cracked. She must have got the same fright I did.

I switched off my radio. I didn't want to miss a word.

'Don't think I don't know that you alter your uniform

when you get to school. Are the rules on dress code too good for you?'

'No!' Sara said. She fired me a dirty look, obviously now realising who the snitch was. 'I didn't,' she protested. 'They've been like this all day.'

'Then why did Jade tell me differently?'

I cringed at that. No one likes a telltale.

'She's a liar!' Sara screamed.

'Don't you call her a liar. I believe her more than I believe you.'

'She's just trying to get me into trouble. It's not fair!'

Whack! Linda slapped her across the side of the head. Sara was either not expecting it or too slow to duck out of the way. She cried out in pain. I winced too. I felt that.

Linda didn't hang around to say anything else. Once she'd stormed out of the room I turned away, not wanting to face her. I only wanted Sara to get a bit of a hard time and hoped it would mean I'd get to eat my dinner downstairs. I didn't want her to get hurt. Besides, it wasn't looking like it had made much difference with Linda. I was still stuck here.

When it came to teatime, as with breakfast, there was a plate missing. This time Sara would go without.

As Arlene and I ate our meagre ham sandwiches in our room the atmosphere was toxic. I could sense the seethe coming from both of them. The paltry sandwich was welcome after a day effectively without food but it was hardly substantial. I craved a proper cooked meal.

We returned our empty plates and I hung around in the kitchen hoping that Linda might say something by way of explanation for the way she had been acting. All she said was, 'Right, everyone upstairs to the bathroom.'

She marched us all, even Lisa, to the toilet. What did she have in mind now?

'Get your nighties. We're all getting ready for bed. I want you all tucked up nice and early so you don't disturb Terry anymore.'

We did as we were told. At bedtime Linda ordered us all to the bathroom. She put the two sisters into the shower first and then Lisa and me. Privacy went out the window. Sometimes Lisa would be in the bath while I was in the shower, as it was in a separate cubicle to the bath in the room that also housed the toilet, a sink and a bidet. There were never any bottles of shampoo, conditioner or shower gel in the shower. Linda dispensed what we needed as and when required.

Tonight Linda lined us all up while she ran a bath for Lisa.

'Arlene, you first,' she said, directing the oldest of us to the shower. It was like a military operation. Linda stood there by the cubicle door, shampoo bottle in hand. She waited until Arlene presented her palm before squirting a ten-pence-piece-sized dollop of shampoo into her palm. I felt sorry for Arlene. She was starting to mature and had more reason to be self-conscious than the rest of us. We didn't know where to look.

'Next,' Linda bellowed to Sara, once Arlene was finished.

I shuffled up the queue until it was my turn.

It was embarrassing, not only to have to stand there naked in front of everyone but also to not be trusted to put on your own shampoo.

As soon as we were all in our nighties and ready for bed, she marched us to the room.

It was still early, around 7 p.m. Surely she didn't expect us to lie in bed until morning? We filed into the bedroom. I looked forward to getting the radio and headphones Dad gave me and listening to some music before we had to go to sleep.

'Right, Arlene, you over there.' Linda pointed to a space on the floor in front of one of the wardrobes. 'Sara, you there.' She was to go over by another wardrobe on the opposite side of the room. 'Jade, you by the bed.' She gestured to the floor by the bunk beds.

'Sit there, all of you. Now, not a sound until it's time for bed.'

My natural instinct was to protest. If Mum tried this I'd have asked what she was on about. Like clockwork, however, both Arlene and Sara dropped to a seating position and sat cross-legged, backs straight, facing away from each other. My position suddenly felt considerably weaker. Feeling like I had no alternative, I slowly lowered myself to the floor.

'A-a-ah,' Linda said, waving a finger, as my bottom hit the carpet.

'What?' I said.

She spun the finger around. 'Face away from the others. Turn your back.'

I saw that Arlene and Sara were facing opposite ends of the room – and then it hit me. That was how they invariably were sitting whenever I'd entered the room before Linda had moved me. This was routine for them. I'd often wondered why they did that. Now I knew. It was years of practice.

I thought about being defiant. Then I remembered how hungry I was and how I didn't want to go another day without food. I leaned against the bed and faced the door, away from the two girls.

'Jade!' Linda said, wagging that same finger. 'No leaning. Back straight.'

I came off the bed frame. In two seconds my back felt stiff.

'Good, now remain like this and there will be no cross words. Goodnight.'

With that she exited the room and closed the door.

I slumped back against the bed. Who the hell did she think she was?

'Jade!'

I nearly jumped from my skin. I hadn't even heard the door squeak open and she was there, filling the frame, silhouetted against the light from the hallway.

'What did I say about slouching?'

'Sorry,' I said, my voice trembling.

I sat up straight, not looking at the others until she closed the door once more. A draught coming in from the old sash window made me shiver. I pulled my knees to my chest and tucked them under my nightie. I had been in the house for over a year now and it was seriously small on me – where once it used to cover my knees, now it stopped at the top of my legs. I looked to the Calor gas heater that might have given the room some warmth, had Linda ever turned it on. I glanced at the other girls. They had not flinched when Linda had burst back in. Even for a second. Nor had they wavered when ordered to sit in their corners. Is that what years of conditioning in the Bad Room did to you? Is that what would happen to me? Was there anything I could do to stop it?

Chapter 11

In the last days of school before we broke up for Christmas I walked around in a daze. I couldn't understand what was happening. Why was Linda persecuting me so much? Did she not want to be my permanent carer?

A contact meeting with Jack and Ellen was arranged for 22 December, with our foster carers and social worker, so we could exchange presents. In front of Shona and the other carers Linda was back to her smiley self. She was like best of friends with Shona, praising me and making no mention of the recent incidents.

'And how are things with you, Jade?' Shona said.

What should I say? Should I tell her about being shut in the Bad Room, going without dinner? The beating? I recalled the previous time Linda hit me, when I'd told my mum and she reported it. Social services might have seemed keen to sweep it under the carpet but Shona had said if it happened again I was to tell her.

I thought about the sort of meeting it would lead to. I could imagine Linda giving her side of the story – how we were unruly, how we needed to be disciplined. No one would believe my side. Linda would make it look like I was only complaining because I wasn't getting my way. Then, when the social worker left, and I was at her mercy, Linda would make my life even more miserable. For that reason I decided I would keep quiet and hope that by doing so it earned me some brownie points with her.

'It's all fine,' I told the social worker.

'That's good to hear,' Shona said, 'because I have news of my own. I'm leaving the council so I'll no longer be your social worker.'

'Oh,' I said. Shona was the social worker I'd liked the most. She'd been a constant presence when everything around me was chaotic.

'I'm sorry. But I will still see you. It won't be as regular as it is now. You'll have other social workers helping you. But I'll arrange to see you every few weeks. Would you like that?'

I nodded and shrugged, trying not to let it show how much her news affected me. It was yet another sign of things changing and all the more reason not to tell her what had been happening. She was leaving. She wouldn't be able to do anything anyway.

I tried to put it all to the back of my mind and concentrate on having fun with my brother and sister. As always it was great to see them. Ellen was getting big and becoming a real handful. She was living with Sally now and I was happy to catch up with her too. My contact sessions with my siblings were the only family time I had now. The meetings with my dad had dried up, with no explanation why, and I hadn't heard from Mum since she'd gone into hospital to have her baby. It seemed like everything was changing. We were approaching a new millennium; some people were getting excited about it, but all I had was a sense of unease.

In the run-up to Christmas Day, though, the house was a bit more of a relaxed place. Linda was more her usual self. Terry was off work, so that might have had something to do with it.

On Christmas morning we were all allowed downstairs. We opened what presents we had and played with any new toys and games. It was fun hanging out with Lisa again and I almost forgot how miserable I'd been in the run-up to the school holidays. Linda's family came round for dinner and we ate together and played games. Rebecca and Deborah always seemed pleased to see me and for those few hours I felt like I was part of a normal family again.

At night we all had to line up, military style, for our showers but Linda had allowed us to stay up a bit later and for the first time in ages I went to bed feeling satisfied, having had a hearty meal. Nevertheless we didn't want to incur Linda's wrath, so we kept the noise down. We didn't want to give her a reason to be mad. Plus an atmosphere still existed between the two sisters and me. We didn't trust each other. Just because we were cooped up in that room together didn't mean we were going to be best friends.

After Christmas it was more like it used to be. I could come and go as I pleased, but only within the house. Linda forbade any of us leaving the house, unless it was with her or Terry. That meant I couldn't see any of the friends I'd made at school. I didn't have a mobile phone and we weren't allowed to use the landline, so the only way for my friends to meet me was to call in. A couple of times I heard them come to the door. Linda said I wasn't allowed out so I had to sit there while she told them I wasn't available. On one occasion I don't think she knew I could overhear her when she said I wasn't in because I was at my dad's. I wanted to shout out of the window, 'I'm here. Don't go,' but it was no use. I wasn't allowed out and she never let friends in the house. It was deeply frustrating but there was nothing I could do about it.

At least I could play with our new games and got to watch TV with Lisa or play on her consoles. It was a return to how it had been when I first arrived. I started to think Linda must have been stressed when she was being mean to us. It had been a phase, similar to when she'd just got out of hospital. Maybe she hadn't been feeling well again and had taken it out on us. Whatever the reason, it was over and we could relax a bit. Life had improved so much in the house that I asked if I could go back into Lisa's room. Since Linda had moved back into her bedroom and the Ukrainian girls had left there had been a spare bunk in her daughter's room. I missed being able to watch TV with Lisa and play on her games consoles. Now we were all on better terms again, could we go back to that arrangement?

'No,' Linda said bluntly. 'It's easier if you girls are all together in that room and we might have to take in a new child at some point in the future so it's best to have the space available.'

I was gutted. Even though things had improved I'd do anything to get out of that room. Still, New Year's Eve was approaching and Linda said she was having their family around again for a party to welcome in the new millennium. That would be good, I thought: another chance to hang out with Rebecca and Deborah and stay up late.

The day passed like the others that holiday, us children kicking about, amusing ourselves, looking forward to the festivities. Come six o'clock Linda called us to the kitchen.

'Upstairs to your room, you three.'

Already, I thought? Maybe, though, we'd be getting a chance to change into nicer clothes for the party.

'I want you out of the way before everyone arrives.'

'What?' I said. 'Already?'

She was deadly serious. 'Is there an issue with that?'

'But it's still early. What about the party?'

Linda's blue eyes flashed. 'That's for the family.'

'That's not fair!' The words were out before I could stop them. I was burning with a sense of injustice.

'I'll show you what's not fair. Get upstairs now!'

'But we haven't had tea.'

'And you can think about that when you're in your room. Get upstairs, now!'

She frogmarched us upstairs and in fifteen minutes we were all showered and shut up in the room with our nighties on.

'Well done, Jade,' Arlene sneered. 'You couldn't keep your big mouth shut.'

'It's not my fault. She was sending us up here anyway,' I said, still fuming at how unfairly we'd been treated. I couldn't believe she was blaming me.

'We might have still got our tea though.'

'What? A sandwich with a pathetic piece of ham?'

'It's better than no food.'

'Maybe if you two spoke up more we wouldn't be in this mess,' I said.

'We've tried that before. We know where that gets you.'

'Stop arguing,' Sara said. 'You're going to make it worse.'

As though on cue, the door swung open. No matter how many times it happened I still got a fright.

'If you three can't stay quiet I'll have to make you. Get on the floor in your corners.'

'But …'

'Do it!' she yelled.

The girls were already on the floor. I reluctantly lowered myself down. So much for Linda being nice again.

When her extended family arrived, it was agony hearing them downstairs having a ball, no doubt stuffing their faces while we languished upstairs. Any thoughts that having her relatives there might mean Linda was less inclined to check on us quickly went out the window when she appeared every few minutes to check we were still in our positions. We'd been like this for a couple of hours when, after she closed the door on us for the umpteenth time that night, I needed to take some action. I had heard what sounded like Lisa going up and down the stairs. I thought if I could get word to her that we were starving she might be able to help.

'What are you doing?' Arlene said when I got to my feet.

'Trying to get us some food.'

'Sit down. You'll get us into more trouble. She's on the warpath.'

'Then blame me. You do all the time anyway.'

'Shut up.'

'Stop it, you two,' Sara said.

They both watched as I edged to the door. There was so much noise of chatter and music from downstairs I figured there was no way Linda would hear the door. My only fear was that she was lurking outside or at the top of the stairs, like I'd seen her do before she trapped me in here.

I gave the handle the firm pull it needed to open. It did so with the usual squeak. I caught my breath. Even with a houseful of guests it sounded like an almighty screech. I heard one of the girls gasp behind me.

'Sssh,' I said, realising that was only adding to the noise we were making.

I slowly opened the door, watching as the shaft of light from the hall widened around the door until I had enough to peek outside. She didn't appear to be right by the door. Good. I opened it a little further. There was no sign of her at the top of the stairs either. I pulled it enough for me to poke my head out.

The noise from downstairs was louder than I thought – a medley of chatter, laughter and music. It was actually so noisy I worried I wouldn't be able to hear the telltale sounds of someone coming. The stairs were such that anyone, even someone as small as Linda, could see if our door was open just by climbing one or two steps.

'Jade!'

Oh my God! I nearly peed my pants. There was someone on the landing. Instinctively I ducked back inside and was about to shut the door when I realised who it was. Lisa. Thank goodness.

'What are you doing?' she said.

'What are *you* doing? You nearly gave me a heart attack.'

'Just getting something from my room. Are you guys not coming down?'

I opened the door wide enough again to see her standing outside the door. 'We're not allowed.'

'Been naughty again?'

'Something like that. Listen, Lisa, can you do us a favour?'

Her eyes narrowed. 'What exactly?'

'I bet there are loads of nice treats down there. Could you get us some please?'

She continued to eye me suspiciously.

'You'll need to be careful so no one sees you. If anyone asks you could be taking a stash to your room. What do you say? Please?!'

'Yeah, okay,' she said brightly, not even pausing to think about it. 'Just some crisps and stuff?'

'That would be magic. Whatever you can get.'

She skipped down the stairs. I was hoping the suggestion of being discreet might make her think it was some sort of game. I closed the door over and took my place on the floor.

'She'll never do it,' Arlene said.

'Yeah she will. You'll see.'

I hoped I was right. If she got caught coming up the stairs the consequences for us could be severe.

An age seemed to pass. Downstairs the chatter continued. There was no sign of Lisa.

'Told you,' Arlene said.

'Give her some time at least,' I said, but inside I had to agree with her. It was probably a stupid idea. As if Lisa would smuggle food into our room, defying her mum in the process.

Just then there was a bump at the door. It swung open and there was Lisa, her hands and arms bursting with Pringles, chocolate fingers, some other biscuits and crisps. We all jumped up and escorted her as she dumped her wares on the table.

'You're a legend. Thank you!'

'Yeah, thanks Lisa,' echoed Arlene and Sara.

'Did you have any bother?' I asked.

'Nah, no one noticed.'

'Think you could get some more?' I said, cheekily. We were already chancing it.

'Sure,' she said.

Lisa made two more successful forays downstairs. For the three hungry girls trapped in the Bad Room it was a godsend. We were so grateful. She sat with us for a little bit, filling us in with what was going on. It was after 10 p.m. and the countdown to midnight and the year 2000 was well under way. When she wanted to go back down-stairs I got her to the door. She'd just stepped onto the landing when I heard voices from the living room.

'Where have the kids been hiding all night anyway?' I heard someone say. I thought it was Rebecca.

'Playing in their room. They didn't want to join us.' That voice was unmistakable – Linda. Liar!

'I'll go get them,' Rebecca said. 'It's a once-in-a-life-time opportunity. They should be down here, playing.'

'No, no,' Linda said. 'I'll go get them.'

'Quick!' I pushed Lisa to go down the stairs and shut the door. As I motioned to Arlene and Sara to get back on the floor I swept any crumbs off the table and plonked myself down. A second later the door swung open.

'Right, come on. Put some clothes on. You can join us downstairs now.'

We didn't need to be told twice. We were up and dressed and downstairs in seconds. It was lovely to see her family, who I always got on with and who clearly were completely oblivious to our treatment. We all stuck to the line that we'd been playing in our room. Our priority, however, was to head to the table where Linda had laid out a buffet of snacks and treats. We stuffed our faces.

As midnight approached we filed into the back garden, where Terry and their sons were about to set off fireworks to celebrate the dawning of the new millennium. We joined in the countdown and let off a big cheer when the clock struck twelve.

Why couldn't it always be like this, I thought, when it was finally time for us to head back upstairs to our beds. There was no need to treat us this way. We weren't naughty kids who needed punishing all the time. We rarely stepped out of line. I had no idea what the new millennium would bring, but any thoughts that it might herald some more happy moments like the New Year celebrations were very quickly dispelled.

Chapter 12

We were two days into the New Year when it happened. I got up on 2 January and went downstairs, had breakfast and looked for the music player that Dad had given me. I was sure I'd left it at the foot of the stairs. It was gone.

'Have you seen my Walkman?' I said to Linda.

'No, dear. Where did you leave it?'

'Right there,' I said, pointing to the bottom of the stairs.

'No. I was tidying some things away this morning but I didn't see it,' she said. 'Are you sure you didn't leave it in the park?'

We had walked to the local park on New Year's Day and I'd taken my Walkman but I definitely brought it back.

'No, I had it in the house.'

'Are you sure? Because I know what you kids are like with losing things.'

I didn't know what that was supposed to mean, as I hardly had any possessions and this was my most prized one. I hunted everywhere for it, asking Lisa and the other girls. It had to be somewhere.

'I think you've left in the park,' Linda said. 'You might be more careful next time.'

I was devastated. I ran to my room and lay on the bed crying to the girls: 'I know I haven't left it in the park because I was listening to it in the house yesterday afternoon.'

I cursed myself for not taking it to the room with me the day before but Linda had marched us upstairs and I forgot to go back and get it. Then we were stuck in the room. It was everything to me – my only source of music, a last link to my dad, who seemed to have disappeared from my life again, and the one thing that made me happy ... an antidote to life in the Bad Room when things got horrible.

That wasn't all.

All of the new presents – the toys and games – we'd received for Christmas were gone. When I asked Linda about those she had an explanation: 'I've removed them. You've played with them enough. It's time to concentrate on going back to school.'

She'd moved them into the dining room, a room they didn't use, except for storage.

'She's done that to us before,' Arlene told me when I complained at the injustice. 'You get to play with them for a few days and then they're gone. At first she said we'd get them back when we learned how to behave – but that was never.'

Without my radio and our new toys, life was unfathomably dull. Now her family had gone and the festivities were over we were back to our confinement in the Bad Room, where all we had to amuse ourselves was the box of Lego and the notepads, pens and pencils.

I felt very alone. With nothing to do all day I sat and moped, my mind working overtime. I tried to think about the good times with Mum. They were so few and far between. Almost always they involved music, but when I remembered dancing on the bed or joining her when she'd get excited when a particular song she loved came on it only made me sadder. Then my thoughts would wander to the bad times, when Paul and she fought like mad, and when I bore the brunt of their fury or frustration. Then I wanted to cry that Mum and Dad couldn't have stayed together for longer. If that had happened Mum wouldn't have met Paul, drugs wouldn't have come into our lives and he wouldn't have made an addict out of her. We'd have had a more settled life and not been in and out of care homes and refuges. That wouldn't have led me to here, with this vindictive, cruel old woman, who had social services wrapped around her finger. Thinking of how events had transpired to land me here made me upset and angry. I wanted to scream at the injustice of it all. How come some children had happy lives and I was stuck in this cold, awful room? It wasn't fair.

It didn't help to dwell on things too long. It wasn't going to change anything and I just had to somehow make the most of this miserable situation. Best to block that stuff out. To try to amuse myself I began drawing. I remembered the advice Mum gave me about how to draw faces so I sketched pictures like I used to do with her, before all the problems started. It helped to while away an hour or so, but on those days before we went back to school time dragged.

Now Terry was back at work we didn't go out and, although he wasn't around to disturb, Linda insisted we stay in our room 'where we couldn't cause any trouble'. The way she spoke you'd think we were three tearaways ripping the house apart. It was torture, just having to sit there. Sometimes I could hear the sound of the TV or the PlayStation coming from Lisa's room and the misery was amplified. Being so close to things that other kids take for granted but not able to use them was excruciating. It wasn't fair on Lisa either. I was sure she'd rather have had someone to play with, but it was like Linda would rather punish her too, to a degree.

I began to see that Terry had no idea what went on in the Bad Room. When he came home, if it coincided with when we happened to be downstairs or heading to the bathroom, he made the odd comment about wondering what we did all day up there. I don't think he knew his wife was capable of treating us so badly. When he was around Linda was sweetness and light, but when he wasn't in earshot she used him as the excuse to mete out all manner of cruelty.

'You need to be quiet so as not to disturb him,' she said, justifying another evening trapped inside those four walls.

I couldn't wait for school to start again. At last I could get out of the house, meet my friends and have some respite from Linda.

In early January a contact meeting was arranged with Jack and Ellen and my new social worker, Claire. She seemed pleasant enough but once again I had to sit there and watch as Linda turned on the charm and made out she was the foster carer of the year. Claire asked me questions about my progress, but in front of Linda. How was I supposed to be able to speak candidly about life in the house with her listening to our every word? Often she answered for me, butting in to say something. All I could do was nod meekly. I didn't want to make things worse than they were.

Yet, even when I said nothing, I was powerless to stop that happening.

I'd only been back at school a few weeks when a friend said to me: 'Is it true you're in foster care?'

I was so shocked I didn't know how to respond. I managed to work out that one girl in my class was going about saying it. I challenged her to tell me who'd told her.

'The girl in the year above who you live with,' she said. 'The one who's also in foster care.'

'What else did she say?'

She looked reluctant but I told her it was better for me to know what was being said.

'That your mum was a drug addict in prison.'

The very last thing I didn't want people to know. I could kill that Sara.

Luckily my friends didn't bother when I explained a little about my situation. I didn't want to tell them everything. I was too embarrassed. At least it wasn't like anyone was picking on me, but I was still furious. What right did Sara have to go around saying that about me? I remembered Linda warning me about her and her saying how harmful it could be to me if it got out. What would Linda make of this if I told her? Was there a chance she might take pity on me and move me out of the Bad Room? There was only one way to find out.

I got home before Sara and immediately sought out Linda to tell her.

'We'll see about this,' she said.

She kept me downstairs until Sara came home, which was only a few minutes later. Linda waited until she'd gone up to the room, then she said, 'Come with me.'

'What?'

'Come on now.'

I immediately got a bad feeling in my stomach. I followed Linda upstairs. We went into the bedroom. Sara was sitting on her bunk.

'Get down here,' Linda said. 'Jade says you've been telling people she's in foster care.'

Sara jumped to the floor and shrugged. 'What's the big deal? She is.'

'You know fine well how children are when they find out something. Jade could be bullied over this.'

Sara said nothing.

'Well, what do you say to Jade?'

She stayed silent.

A slight smile played on Linda's lips.

'Jade, I think you have the right to hit Sara for that.'

'What?' Incredulous, I looked at the foster carer. Sara's expression matched mine.

'Go on, hit her,' Linda said, staring at Sara.

'No!'

'She's spreading stories about you. She deserves it. Hit her!'

Sara looked at me pleadingly. This was crazy. I was annoyed that people knew the truth about me but I wouldn't have hit Sara over it.

'Go on,' Linda insisted. 'Teach her a lesson. We're not leaving here until you do.'

Still I hesitated. I couldn't believe a grown-up was telling a kid to hit another kid. Usually they stepped in to break up fights, not instigate them.

'I don't want to.'

'Yes you do. I could see it in your eyes when you came home. You wanted her to be punished. Well, it's no good me doing it. You need to do it.'

Her eyes flashed between us. She was enjoying this.

'Go on. Hit her!'

'No. I don't want to hit her.'

'Do as you're told or I'll hit you. Do you want that? Or what about if Sara hits you for making up stories about her?'

She had this mad leer on her face. She raised her hand. I didn't know what else to do so I smacked Sara on the arm.

'Ow,' Sara said. 'That hurt.'

Linda started cackling. It was horrible. 'Do it again. Hit her harder!'

'No! Please. That's enough.' I wanted to cry.

Linda looked disappointed.

'Very well then. You two can stew it out in here together. I don't know which one of you is telling the truth so you can both sit in here in silence.'

'But that's not …' I stopped myself before I said too much.

'Not what?' Linda said, her face inches from mine. I could smell stale coffee and cigarettes. I wanted to be sick.

'Nothing,' I mumbled.

'Good,' she said, heading to the door. 'And if I hear any evidence of you two fighting or arguing you'll both go without your tea.'

She slammed the door shut.

I sloped down on the floor, feeling horrible. I didn't feel mad with Sara anymore. I was cross with myself for thinking that Linda would ever try to help me. Something clicked in my head that what just happened wasn't right. She was playing us off each other and revelling in it.

It wasn't long before Arlene came home.

'What's happened?'

Both of us sat in silence. I felt ashamed and didn't want to tell her.

'Linda got Jade to hit me,' Sara said eventually, when Arlene pushed her to tell.

'Why?'

'She told everyone at school I'm in foster care.'

'Did you?' Arlene said to her sister.

She shrugged. 'Everyone knows anyway. It's not like it's a big secret.'

She was probably right. And it hadn't been a big deal. The people I liked had probably suspected anyway and didn't care when I confirmed it.

'I'm sorry I hit you,' I said to Sara.

'And I'm sorry I said that about you.'

We sat in silence for a bit. I thought about the things Linda had said about my roommates.

'Linda said I wasn't to talk to you two,' I said.

'Why?' Sara said.

'She always said you were naughty, that you couldn't be trusted. That's why she has to be so strict.' I felt bad about saying this. 'She says horrible things.'

I told her some of what Linda had told me about them.

'She's such a liar,' Sara said.

Arlene just stared at the floor. I wasn't sure if she was seething mad or about to cry. 'She's said stuff to us about you too.'

'What sort of stuff?' Now it was my turn to feel mad.

They looked at each other as though deliberating whether to tell.

'What?' I said, my blood boiling.

'Also horrible stuff,' she said, going on to say things that sounded strangely familiar.

'That's exactly what she says about you!' I was livid. How could someone be so mean? 'Why does she say that stuff?'

Sara sighed. 'I don't know. It's not true. She just lies about everything.'

'What even happened to you two?' I asked. 'Why are you in here?'

They exchanged looks again before Arlene spoke. 'Something happened at home and social services said our mum and dad weren't able to look after us anymore.'

'Do you ever see them?'

'We used to,' Arlene said. 'When we first came here we got to see our mum and dad. We've got another sister and we saw her too. Then the meetings stopped. We've not seen them for ages.'

'That's what happened to me.' I told them my story, how we came to end up in care and how I hadn't seen my mum or dad in a while.

'That's what Linda does,' Arlene said. 'For the first year or so it's great. She makes it seem fun here, a better place to live, and then once she's convinced social services that everyone's happy she turns.'

'Why, though?' I said.

They shrugged.

'Why give your home to children if you don't like them being here?'

'For money?' Arlene said. 'She gets paid for every child she gives a home to. Plus money for lunches, clothes, toys. We should get everything that social services gives her, but we don't.'

'It's not fair,' I said. That was the one thought that was going through my head. This. Is. Not. Fair.

I put my back against the bed and groaned. We sat like this for what seemed an eternity. Under Linda's rules we weren't allowed to go to the toilet other than when she told us we could go. We also had to wait until she called us when our tea was ready. I had been listening out for the call but none came. I was sure I could hear Lisa going down for her meal. Still there was no call.

'Should we not have had tea by now?'

Arlene shrugged. 'Maybe,' Sara said.

'I'm going to investigate.'

'If she catches you then you're definitely going without,' Arlene said. She was always the most negative.

'Looks like that's what's happening anyway.'

I went to the door and did the customary check to listen for any obvious signs. Noise of Linda talking loudly downstairs was always the most reassuring sound. I opened the door, stepped out onto the landing and peered down the stairs. There on the bottom step were three plates. Incredibly, it was fish fingers and chips. It was so rare that she could be bothered to cook for us these days. I ducked back inside.

'She's left the food out. It's fish fingers!'

They both leapt to their feet.

'Wait,' Arlene said. 'She's not called for us. We'll get into trouble if we go down.'

'But what if she has and we haven't been down? We'll lose it anyway?' Sara said.

'I'm not hanging about to find out.' I ran downstairs and was about to pick up a plate when Linda appeared out of the kitchen.

'What do you think you're doing?'

'Getting my tea.'

'No you don't.'

'What?' I looked to see where Arlene and Sara were. They were lingering at the top of the stairs.

'It's cold now. I called ages ago but you obviously weren't hungry – or were too busy talking or arguing to hear me. You've ruined it now – so you will go without.'

'No! Please, I don't care if it's cold. I'll eat it,' I said reaching again for the plate.

'Get your hands off. You had your chance, Jade. Now you can think some more about how you behave.'

I reached for another of the plates but she was too fast, scooping them all up and taking them back through to the kitchen. Tears were welling up in my eyes and I watched in disbelief as she opened the bin and scraped the food away.

'It's not fair!' I yelled, turning and running up the stairs. Arlene and Sara were already in the room. They seemed to be far more accepting of their supposed 'punishment'.

'She was never going to give us it,' Arlene said. 'She didn't call us down on purpose.'

Fury threatened to consume me. I wanted to hit something, anything, to expel the burning injustice.

I barely heard the squeak of the door before a stiff slap on the arm sent me tumbling onto the bed. Linda had burst into the room. I tried to grab the duvet but I was yanked backwards, off the bed and onto the floor. I caught sight of a black leather boot as it made contact with my leg. I was too shocked to yell out and still trying to get a sense of what was happening.

'Don't you complain to me about "not fair",' Linda hissed in my ear. 'Not fair is me slaving to make you ungrateful brats a nice dinner and you ignoring me. You can stay seated on the floor in your positions for a bit longer!'

I cowered, trying to make myself as small as possible, tucking my legs up and covering my head in case of any more blows. There were none. I lifted my head in time to see Linda make for the door.

'I need the toilet,' I whimpered.

'Tough. And that goes for all of you.' She waved a bony finger around all three of us.

She switched off the light and slammed the door shut.

The shock wore off, quickly replaced by pain. My whole body was shaking. 'It's not fair,' I whispered, over and over as I tried to compose myself.

In the darkness I sensed two pairs of eyes boring into me. It was going to be a long night.

Chapter 13

'Good going, Jade.' The whispered voice in the darkness could only have been Arlene, but having just
opened my eyes they had yet to adjust and it was hard
to make out her features. I imagined she was glaring at
me though.

'How is it my fault?'

'You got her angry.'

'What?' I'd been going over that evening's events
several times in my head, trying to make sense of it all.
'If anything it was Sara's fault for spreading stories
about me.'

'You didn't have to tell Linda.'

'It's not my fault she wanted me to hit her. She's the
one to blame, not me.'

'We could have got our tea if you hadn't run down
the stairs.'

'Maybe if you backed me up she wouldn't think she
could get away with not feeding us. You just sit there
and take it.'

That wasn't entirely true. Arlene was generally quiet and didn't get involved but there had been times, like when Lisa told stories about who she was hanging around with at their school, when she lost it. And when Arlene lost it she really went mental. I could swear even Linda was scared sometimes. Arlene was taller than her and I was sure if she put her mind to it she could give Linda quite a fright. For the most part, she shied away from confrontation. I don't know how they did it. I'd only been in this room for a few weeks and already it was driving me mad. They'd been dealing with it for years.

'I know what she's like. There's no point arguing. It only makes it worse.'

She had a point there. Linda never needed an excuse to punish us. Since she'd told us to sit on the floor she'd paid us intermittent visits, claiming she could hear us talking or had caught one or more of us moving position, which she said earned us half an hour extra each time. We'd now been sitting like this, in the dark, for hours. My back and bottom were stiff from being in the same position, my tummy was rumbling and my leg was sore from where she had kicked me. Given half a chance I'd have happily retrieved the fish fingers from the bin and eaten them, I was that hungry.

'Will you two keep it down? I want to go to bed. At this rate she'll keep us up all night like this.'

I hadn't heard from Sara for a while. I actually thought she'd nodded off.

'Tell your sister to shut up then – and stop blaming me,' I said.

'So it's my fault, is it?' Arlene said.

'Please. Just keep it down!'

A bright flash of light into the room had us all blinking and shielding our eyes. Linda must sneak up the stairs as she always managed to burst in without warning.

'You three find it impossible to do what you're told.' She stood in the middle of the room pointing at us. 'Jade, was that you being naughty again?'

'No!'

Her face, lit up by the light from the hallway, took on a sinister leer. She raised her hand as if to hit me again. I braced myself for another assault.

'Who was it then?'

'Sara!' Her name was out before I thought of the implications.

'I thought as much.'

Linda swivelled and lunged for Sara where she sat in front of one of the wardrobes. She swung and slapped her on the head. Her victim flinched and fell to the floor but did nothing to shield herself. She just lay there. Linda momentarily looked as though she wasn't sure what to do next, but then she strode over and kicked her leg. She knelt down and whacked her a third time on the side of arm. Again, Sara just lay there. I was willing her to defend herself. Linda kicked out again with a large boot.

'Stop it!' Arlene shouted. She was up on her knees but still in front of her wardrobe.

Linda turned, arm raised again.

'Do you need a telling too?'

Arlene cowered back. 'No, just leave her alone.'

'Right ...' Linda strode around the middle of the room as though trying to work out her next move, '... that's enough. If you keep on with this noise you'll keep Terry awake and he has to be up before the crack of dawn. All of you get to your beds now.'

Sara continued to lie there on her side on the floor.

'Please,' Arlene said. 'Can I go to the toilet? I'm bursting.'

'Well, that's your problem. That's why you need to behave when you come home from school. You only have yourselves to blame.'

'But I'll wet the bed!'

'If you want to go to school stinking like a filthy scrubber that's up to you.'

'But please. We've not been able to go since we came home.'

'That's your problem.' With that Linda turned and left. The door closed, returning the room to darkness.

Sara got up slowly. She appeared to be wincing but climbed up to her bunk.

'Are you okay?' I whispered.

'Yes, but my head hurts.'

I was desperate to go to the toilet but I knew from watching Linda's behaviour when I wasn't in the room that it was those moments after she'd left that she most expected to catch us out.

We all got changed into our nighties. Every movement made my bladder hurt. If I didn't leave soon to go to the toilet I'd have an accident. I crept towards the door.

'What are you doing?' It was Sara.

'I need to go to the toilet. I'm bursting.'

I could barely move. It was agony to stand up straight and if I bent over the relief was almost too much to contain. I got to the door. My discomfort was so intense I couldn't concentrate hard enough to know if there were sounds from another part of the house. I was so desperate I just had to go and suffer any consequences. Anything was better than the current state I was in.

'We all need to go. You'll make it worse for all of us,' hissed Arlene.

'Shut up!' I struggled to keep my voice down. My eyes were watering. The pain was excruciating. I pulled at the door with my right hand, left over my bladder, bent over like a little old lady. The door wouldn't budge. I could see the latch move but it was held by something. What made this door stick so much? I gave it a yank and the door let out an almighty screech, ten times louder than normal.

'Jade!' Sara said, a little too loudly.

'Shut the door!' Arlene said. 'Quick, before she comes.'

I wasn't listening to them. I only had one thought in my mind. Get to the toilet. Nothing else mattered. The light from the landing hurt my eyes. The pain in my stomach was unbearable. I tried to put a hand to shield my eyes but I needed it to feel my way along the wall, as I couldn't stand upright. I needed my other hand on my bladder. To move it would mean catastrophe. I was vaguely aware of noises downstairs but everything was a blur. Linda could have been standing right behind me and I wouldn't have registered. I had to make it to the bathroom. It was at the end of the landing, only a few steps away normally but in the state I was in it felt like ten miles away. I shuffled along, every ounce of my being crying out to relieve myself. Tiny steps took me past Lisa's door. I didn't even know if she was in her room. I had no idea what time it was. Only the lights on upstairs told me that at least one person was still up. It could be midnight for all I knew. This whole afternoon had been so weird, the confrontation with Sara after school felt like weeks ago.

I could see the bathroom door. I was still bent over, shuffling slowly along the landing, but it was getting closer. I couldn't help imagining how good it would feel to have done my business and be back to normal. It would be so nice to be lying in bed free of this discomfort. The pain in my leg and arm I couldn't even feel now. This had taken over everything. I was almost there. Just a few more steps and I'd be inside the bathroom. There I could lock the door and take all the time I wanted. It would be bliss. I couldn't care if Linda caught me. Nothing she could do would be worse than this.

I shuffled the last couple of steps and put my hand on the door knob. I could see from the dark around the door that no one was inside. I hadn't even given consideration to the fact that it could be occupied. I pushed open the door and edged inside. There was the toilet. Thank God.

I almost felt well enough to stand up. I'd made it. I turned to push the door shut behind me. And that's when I saw the boots.

'Where the hell do you think you're going?'

The fright almost brought on the leak I'd been trying so hard to avoid. No! Not when I had made it this far. I actually tried to push the door shut but it jarred against her boot. I didn't have the energy to push again. I turned and reached for the toilet. I'd do it anyway. Screw her.

A hand grabbed my arm and pulled me towards the door.

'Please. I'm bursting. My tummy hurts. Please let me go.'

'I told you to stay in your room.'

'But I'll wet myself.'

She pulled me more firmly.

'If that's the only way you'll learn to listen to me in future, then so be it.'

Willing my bare feet to stick to the tiled bathroom floor, I summoned all the strength I had to resist her attempt to pull me back. With her hand under my armpit she yanked me upright. And then it happened. Being forced to stand broke some kind of hold I had on my bladder and the waters broke. Warm liquid ran down my leg onto the bathroom floor. I let out a moan, part joy and part utter embarrassment. I couldn't remember the last time I'd had an accident. Suddenly I regained my conscious self. The fuzzy brain feeling had gone. I just wanted the ground to swallow me up. And I knew I was for it now.

'You disgusting creature. Is this how you were raised? To do the toilet anywhere you like?'

Linda still gripped hold of my arm, her fingers pressing into my flesh. Oh the relief when it was over. For a split second I almost didn't care. The feeling of ease on my bladder and stomach was worth it. Instinctively I pulled towards the sink. I obviously needed to get cleaned up.

'Where are you going?'

'To wash myself.'

Her grip tightened. 'Oh no you don't.'

With strength that belied her stature, she dragged me out of the bathroom and back along the landing. The journey back took a fraction of the time it had taken me to get there, my feet frantically trying to keep up with her giant strides. She battered through the door of the room and pushed me inside. In the half-light I could Sara's eyes blinking to see what was going on. Arlene was pretending to be asleep.

'Stand there,' Linda said pushing me into the middle of the room. 'Take off your filthy soiled clothes.'

'My nightie's okay,' I said, patting myself down. 'It's only really my …'

'Take everything off!' she yelled.

I slipped out of my clothes, flicked the little pile to one side and stood there shivering. It was the middle of January and winter nights in that heat-starved room were icy at the best of times. My legs felt wet and sticky, my nostrils filled with the smell of stale urine. I surely didn't stink that much. Then I twigged. Mine hadn't been the only accident.

'It smells disgusting in here,' Linda said. 'All of you are disgusting.'

'I'm sorry. I couldn't help it,' Sara said. 'I hadn't been all night.'

'And who's fault is that? Eh?!'

'Have you wet the bed as well?' She shook the quilt-covered body of Arlene. She didn't answer. 'Pathetic, all of you.'

'Can I get clean clothes please?' I said, aware that my lips were chilled and my teeth would soon be chattering.

'No.' Her voice was almost calm. She looked like she was pondering something. 'You can stay there, like that, all night. I don't want a dirty little scrubber like you dirtying my clean bed. Stand there until you've learned your lesson that it's not wise to ignore what I say.'

'Please. I'm sorry. I just want to go to bed. I have learned my lesson. Please.'

'Shut up. Just stand there. I'll be checking. If you so much as move an inch there will be no breakfast or lunch for you tomorrow. Do you understand?'

If I hadn't been shivering so much I might have cried. I wrapped my arms tightly around myself and shifted on the balls of my feet, hoping the slight movement might generate some heat. I'd only been standing like this for a couple of minutes and already I was freezing. All night? I would die of hypothermia.

'If I find you've been in bed or have lain on the floor or have got some clean clothes I swear to God you will not know what's hit you, young lady. Now, will this be the end of it?' She spun round addressing our bunks. 'You've all been a disgrace today – hitting each other, arguing, talking, mucking around and wasting your dinner. Wait until social services hear about all this. You'll be in big trouble.'

None of us answered. I assumed we were all feeling completely done in – hungry, cold and wet. At least Arlene and Sara had a bed to find a dry space in. As the room returned to darkness when she finally exited the room, I weighed up my options. My knees were knocking together, keeping a different rhythm to my teeth. I rubbed my hands against the tops of my arms but they did little to stave off the shivers. I stood for what seemed like an age. All around me was silence, save for the gentle breathing from the two beds. They were asleep. I had to do something to try to join them.

Lowering myself to the floor, I hugged my legs. They were like icicles. I curled into a ball and pulled my discarded nightie over me like the thinnest make-shift blanket. It barely covered my body but it was a godsend compared to standing in the draught from the window. If she came in I'd have to spring to my feet. I probably wouldn't manage it and she'd hit me once more, or make good on her threats to starve me tomorrow.

In that moment, though, I didn't care. I wanted to cry. For the misery of it all, for not having my radio, for feeling that I'd lost the last remaining link to my dad, for being stuck here in this horrible room. The tears wouldn't even come. I was too tired. Mostly I just wanted to sleep and hope that somehow I would wake up and find that this was all a bad dream.

Chapter 14

I've never spent a more fitful night. Every time I woke up I sprang to my feet in case Linda walked in. Then I realised it was still the dead of night, the rest of the house was asleep and I could curl up on the floor under my nightie, soiled from lying against my legs. Even the nights when Mum had kept me awake were pleasant compared to this.

By the time the girls stirred I was back on my feet, standing there, shivering, facing the other way, praying that Linda would enter soon to see how obedient I'd been and to put me out of my misery. Eventually she did and almost appeared disappointed that I'd done what she'd told me. That didn't stop her from punishing me further, though. She let me go to the bathroom but not to have a shower. It was my fault that I'd not been able to have a shower the night before, so I could 'suffer the consequences'. Using the bidet I cleaned myself as best I could but all through school that day I couldn't escape the smell. I was sure everyone else could smell it and any time anyone made reference to a stench or pong I panicked, convinced they were talking about me. Mercifully, Linda had left out my cereal, so I had eaten standing by the kitchen counter as usual, before picking up my lunch and heading out. At least I wasn't as hungry as I had been, but although I wanted the school day to end so I could clean up, I dreaded going home. What would she find to go nuts about today?

'Let's not have a repeat of yesterday, so to prove to me that you can do as you're told, let's have you sitting on the floor in silence until teatime, okay?' she said when we were all back in the room. 'Right, Arlene, you over there. Sara, you there. Jade, you there. Face away so you can't look at each other and there's no temptation to talk or make faces or use sign language.'

Was she serious? Sign language? We got into our positions. She made sure we weren't close enough to the beds or wardrobes. We just had to sit there, facing the walls. In an attempt to distract us from any mischief she said we could have our notepads to draw in. We had no choice but to go along with it. If we played the game we might get our dinner.

I tried to use the time constructively, sketching in the pad like the way Mum taught me. Taking only the odd glance round at the others I saw that Sara was building something from some of the Lego, while Arlene just looked like she was lost in her own little world. None of us spoke. None of us dared. We'd been like that for the entire time we'd spent in the room since coming home from school.

After finishing one sketch I tore out the paper and tossed it to one side. Probably due to the draught from the window, it floated over to where Sara was. She saw it and picked it up.

'That's really good,' she said, half whispering, half mouthing. She floated it back over towards me. It flipped up in the air and looked like it was going to land back by her feet when a gust of air blew it in my direction. The door had swung open. There she was, in her customary black boots, hair up, bright blue eyes scanning the room, no doubt looking for some minor misdemeanour she could punish us for.

'Who's been talking?'

We all looked at her, incredulously. Did she really hear those few whispered words from Sara? If so she must have been outside the door straining to hear for any indiscretion, or she was chancing it, imagining that we must be up to something. I wouldn't put either past her.

'No one,' I said, remaining calm.

'Arlene? Tell me. I heard someone talking? Who was it?'

Arlene just stared at the floor.

'Tell me. You don't want to miss out on your tea again.'

Please Arlene, I thought, don't land us in it on the basis of one tiny comment.

'Well …?' Linda paced around, scanning everything, trying to see if there was anything else she could get us on. We hadn't been talking, weren't leaning, hadn't moved. She was trying to play us off each other. She probably had been hiding behind the door waiting for the moment to strike. Now she wanted to see if Arlene would hang one of us to save herself. Surely she wouldn't dob in her own sister for that? If she didn't, that meant she might pick on me instead.

Arlene shook her head. 'No one was speaking.'

'I must have been imagining it then, was I?' Linda's boots squelched as she crouched down to Arlene's level.

The older girl shrugged. 'I didn't hear anyone speaking.'

We all sat there, waiting for the dark cloud to pass over us. No one moved. Surely even she would see that we were playing the game?

'Very well,' she said. She hovered for a bit as though waiting for something. Did she expect Arlene to suddenly shout, 'It was Jade!' Whatever she was doing she obviously thought better of it as she walked out the room and closed the door behind her. As she did so something fell from above where the latch was. It looked like a bit of paper. I was tempted to get up and have a look but experience taught me this was the most dangerous time – just after she left us. We all resumed what we were doing and kept a keen ear out for any signs it was teatime.

It took about half an hour but finally the call came.

'Jade! Your tea's ready!'

This was a very good sign that we were all getting our dinner. My mouth was already salivating at the thought of the fish fingers we'd missed out on the night before. The set-up, if we weren't being punished for something, was the same as I had seen it when I shared Lisa's room, in that she called us one by one to collect our plates to eat in the Bad Room. I raced downstairs, excited to be first. Then I stopped. There were no fish fingers, no chips, no anything that resembled a meal. All that was there was a small plate with two tea biscuits. In between them was one wafer-thin slice of ham. A biscuit sandwich. She had got to be kidding. That was our tea?

'Is there a problem?' Linda was at the foot of the stairs, probably about to call one of the others.

'No. Thank you.'

My pace back upstairs resembled a condemned prisoner. If I'd started eating it now it wouldn't have lasted to the top step. I held up the plate to Sara to show her what she could expect as the call rang out for her to go down. Her face fell too.

Dinner was so underwhelming I went to investigate the paper that fell from the door. It was a solid piece of folded paper.

'What's this?' I said when Arlene came back.

'Just a piece of toilet paper Linda puts in the door to keep it shut.'

I closed and opened the door. No squeak. Interesting. I was going to try to force it back into the space between the door and frame but decided against it and kicked it under the bed. The door still closed over but didn't stick as before.

I ate my biscuit sandwich and then I volunteered to take the plates down. The smell from the kitchen suggested Linda and her family had enjoyed something cooked. I was still hungry and thirsty. The biscuits in no way filled me up but they had succeeded in drying my mouth so it felt like sandpaper. I couldn't ask Linda for a drink. Sometimes she'd give us a small drink with our tea but mostly she hated us drinking in the evening as she said it would make us go to the toilet, which would keep Terry awake. I hoped I might have time to nip to the toilet and drink from the tap but that plan was scuppered when Linda appeared from the living room and called up the stairs: 'Right, shower time.'

We endured the ritual bathroom session, taking it in turns to wash in front of everyone else. By the time I was ready for bed my throat was parched. I had to get a drink. Linda made sure we were all in bed and then closed the door. So far she hadn't noticed the paper had come out of the door. I waited a long time until I was sure she would be watching television downstairs and then I made my move.

I slipped out of bed and crept to the door. I was getting used to the areas of the floor that creaked the most. There was a floorboard just to the left of the door as you approached that always let out a loud groan. I avoided it and headed towards the door. I turned and as expected Sara and Arlene were watching me. Using sign language I tilted a cupped hand to my mouth. Sara pulled her quilt up to her chin.

I felt a bit like a safe cracker when they make their final calculations before going for it. I pulled on the handle. The door gave way with ease. It practically glided open in complete silence. Bliss! I opened it enough to listen to the sounds of the house. Almost instantly Linda's loud laugh could be heard from the living room, along with Terry's. That was a good sign. She'd hardly want to pull herself from the telly if they were watching something funny. Now was my chance. I slipped along the landing. Suddenly the floor creaked. Why had I not noticed that before? I moved my foot but it creaked again. Damn. It was like the whole centre of the floor was primed to give me away. I paused mid-step, holding my position while I checked if Linda had heard. I could still make out the faint sound of the TV. Come on, come on. Laugh again. I imagined her doing the same thing, perched on the dining chair, cigarette in hand. Maybe she was willing me to take another step. Go on, hang yourself. Take one more step. I dare you.

I couldn't believe I hadn't noticed the floor was this creaky. Clearly when I'd tried this before I'd had my mind on other things.

And then there it was. More laughter. Both her and Terry. They clearly found something funny. I took a few more steps, stepping over towards the walls where I was relieved to find the floorboards were kinder. I slipped quietly along, got to the bathroom and got inside.

I ran the tap and gulped down the water as appreciatively as if I'd just trekked for three days across the desert. It didn't matter that the water ran lukewarm for a few seconds before it chilled. I was so grateful for moisture for my parched mouth. I wiped my face and headed back to the room, retracing my steps so as not to make a racket. I got to the top of the landing and was almost going to pause before I crossed the top of the stairs. I heard more laughter, however, and realised I was safe. I slipped into the room, eased the door shut, dodged the problem floorboard and made it into bed.

Immediately I dived under the covers and pulled the quilt around me, expecting the door to burst open and Linda to start yelling. For a few minutes though there was nothing. I poked my head out of the covers and took a deep breath. The sense of achievement was amazing. I'd done it. I'd sneaked out of the room and back in without her realising. I wanted to shout out, I was so happy.

Then it hit me. The bit of paper she jammed in the door. When she eventually discovered it wasn't in place she'd know something had gone on. I needed to put it back.

Slipping out of bed, I got down on the floor and, being careful not to tread on the creaky floorboard, I felt around under the bed for the bit of paper. The carpet was all dusty. I shuddered to think what my hand was raking through to find it. Linda rarely cleaned this room. If she came in now I'd have a lot of explaining to do. My hand found something. It was the bit of paper. It was rock hard and from what I could see in the darkness it had moulded into the shape of the doorframe. No wonder it stayed there for days.

'What are you doing?' It was Sara, peering down from her top bunk.

'Need to put the paper back?' I held it up to show her.

'You're mad! Get to bed,' she whispered.

'Shush.'

I got up and made it to the door without protests from the floorboard. I eased the door open again, shoved the paper in and closed the door. It didn't squeak but it seemed to hold the door in place. I turned to go back to bed.

'Not there.' It was Arlene. She was shaking her head vigorously. 'She puts it higher than that.'

Now I was really chancing it. I didn't want to open the door again in case it squeaked like before and sent Linda charging up. But if Arlene was right I was landing us right in it. I reached for the handle. Like the safe cracker once more, I made my calculations. Slowly but steady, not yanking it too much.

What was that? Someone was coming up the stairs. I heard Linda calling something to Terry but I couldn't make out if it was her coming up or him. I couldn't risk her opening the door and finding me here. Disregarding all precautionary tactics I practically bounded across the floor, leapt into bed and dived under the covers.

The room filled with light. It was Linda.

I peered above the covers, as though her entrance had disturbed me from the deepest sleep. I saw her standing in the doorway, just as the bit of paper fell out and landed at her feet. She stooped and picked it up, holding it out into the light of the landing to inspect it.

'This has been moved.'

How could she tell?

'What have you lot been up to?'

'Uh, what?' I said, doing my best bleary-eyed impression. 'We've not done anything. We've all been in bed.'

'You have been up to something. Sara, what's been going on?'

I heard movement above me.

'Jade got up to go to the toilet.'

I couldn't believe it. The joy I'd felt only moments before turned to horror.

'Did she now?'

'I'm sorry, I only went to get a drink. I was really thirsty.'

She strode over to the bed, hand raised. That was all I saw for I dived down, pulling the quilt around me for protection as the blows came.

'I. Told. You. Not. To. Get. Up.' A smack for every word. 'How am I going to get you to do as I say?'

I wasn't going to poke my head out to give her an answer. I remained curled as tightly as I could.

'This is not over.'

She must have stormed out of the room for it returned to darkness. I stuck my head out for some air and stretched my aching limbs. She'd caught me on the legs and bottom mostly. It could have been worse.

'Thanks, Sara,' I whispered.

'Sorry,' a small voice said.

I slumped back on the pillow, dejected. My mind played over potential punishments that were coming my way. Going without food, being forced to stand up naked for hours? I had no way of knowing. The only thing of which I could be certain was that it would happen – and it would be brutal.

Chapter 15

It's hard to describe what being deprived of food does to you. It's not just the hunger pains. They're bad enough. It's what it does to your brain. You flit from feeling like you have zero energy to being almost manic. The sounds, sights and smells of other people eating when you can't and haven't for hours is torture.

As I'd suspected, there was no breakfast waiting for me the following morning and no lunch either. At school I covered up Linda's cruelty by lying to friends about my situation.

'Oh, she forgot this morning,' I said when they asked why I had no lunch. The truth was too embarrassing. It was bad enough people knowing I was in foster care. I didn't want them to think that was only the start of my suffering. These were friends to whom I'd said, 'It's not that bad,' when they'd asked what living with another family was like. I didn't want them to think it was as grim as they feared, worse even. And the last thing I wanted was their pity.

By the afternoon on days when Linda refused to feed me I was all over the place. It was impossible to concentrate in class. I was irritable and nauseous. I just wanted to get out of there but at the same time dreaded going back to that house. Stuck in the Bad Room there were moments when I felt like a caged animal. I wanted to rebel against this horrible regime so much that I almost didn't care about the consequences.

It took an incredible amount of will power to last until teatime, when I hoped Linda would have grown bored with punishing me and give me something to eat. I wasn't surprised when she called Sara first and then Arlene down for their plates. I was excited to see she'd cooked a frozen pizza. My taste buds started dancing at the prospect. By the time Arlene came back upstairs I was jumping on the spot with excitement.

No call came. I was tempted to leave the room and peek down to see if my plate was there but I knew Linda might view that as disobedience and remove it so I forced myself to stay put. I'd lasted this long. I glanced round at my roommates. Not only were they not making eye contact but they had turned their backs to me. Now that I thought of it, Sara had looked a bit sheepish when she came up the stairs. The pair of them were hunched over their plates as though embarrassed to be eating in front of me.

'There is a plate for me down there, isn't there?'

Sara looked at Arlene before turning to me. 'Sorry,' she said quietly.

'You're joking!'

I couldn't hold back any longer. From the top of the stairs I could see there was no plate. My punishment continued. Sloping back into the room I slumped on the bed. I wanted to cry but I honestly didn't think I could summon any tears even if I wanted to.

Sara glanced over but turned away sharply when our eyes made contact. She must have been feeling guilty for telling on me.

'Could you give me a piece ... please?'

Part of me hated asking and wanted to be tough, to show that I could cope without anyone's charity, but overwhelmingly I was so hungry I could have bitten her arm off.

She turned back but couldn't look me in the eye.

'I can't. I'm sorry,' she whispered. 'She told us not to.'

'How's she going to know?'

Sara shrugged. 'Don't know, but she will.'

I pulled at my hair and fell onto my bed. Torture didn't even come close to this. I told myself not to look but I couldn't help it. And even though they tried to turn away from me I could taste the cheese and tomato, my mouth salivating at their every bite.

When they finished and their plates were empty it set me off again as though yet further confirmation that

I wouldn't be getting anything, not even a mouthful. Arlene gathered the plates to take down but before she left the room Linda appeared.

'I hope you didn't give her any.'

They both shook their heads.

'Let me check. Stand up, Jade.'

What was she on about? I did as I was told. She grabbed my face and yanked open my mouth, sniffing and looking inside.

'It doesn't look like you have. They must like you less than I thought.'

'Ugh, get off,' I said, pushing her hand away. I knew that wouldn't go down well but I couldn't bear her touching me. My own mother wouldn't do such a thing so why should she?

Linda just laughed, though, which made me even madder. She left the room and even though there was a good chance she was waiting outside for me to react in some way I took the opportunity when Arlene carried their plates down to sneak to the toilet for a drink of water. It was reckless but I didn't see her lurking and could hear sounds of her washing up in the kitchen. Even though, I still took care not to make needless noise. I gulped as much water as I could from the tap and snuck back to the room. I'd barely sat down on my bed when Linda appeared.

'Been in the toilet again when you weren't supposed to be?'

How did she know? Had the girls told on me again? I shot them a dirty look for good measure.

'I needed a drink. I'm dying of thirst.'

'You know the rules. After your shower you will stand in the corner until you learn not to disobey them.'

It was all I could do to stop myself crying while we had our showers; both from despair at my situation and anger that she could treat people like this and get away with it.

While Arlene and Sara got ready to climb into their beds I had to stand in the corner. Before she went to bed, though, Arlene came over to me. What did she want? I partly blamed them for my predicament. Was she going to rub salt in my wounds?

'She can hear the taps are on in the kitchen. The pipes, like the toilet flush. She can tell.'

Stunned that she was giving me friendly advice, I also felt stupid. How had I not noticed that? Of course, whenever the toilet was flushed or the taps switched on the water ran down pipes. You could hear it downstairs, particularly in the kitchen. That's how she knew I'd been in the bathroom. If I was going to outwit her I needed to be smarter.

It must have been after 10 p.m. and nearly three hours of standing in the cold, in my nightie, when Linda finally said I could go to bed. I was beyond shattered. I crawled into bed and hardly had the strength to pull my quilt over me. I endured a broken night's sleep, woken at regular intervals by my groaning tummy.

When morning came, although it was dark when I opened my eyes, I was surprised to see the room was empty. Where were Arlene and Sara? I heard noises by the front door. Arlene and Lisa were leaving to go to their school. What time was it?

I got up, quickly got dressed and went to investigate.

'Slept in did you? Lazy madam,' Linda said when I opened the door and saw her at the foot of the stairs.

'What time is it?'

'Time you should be in school. Sara is already away.'

Panic set in. I got my stuff together and raced for the door.

'Not taking your lunch?' Linda said, a weird smile on her face. She must have planned this. She could have woken me. It was her fault I had been awake half the night. I was half amazed to see she'd actually made me lunch but partly annoyed that I had to halt my departure to go and get it.

The streets had that horrible empty feeling when you're late for school and all the children have gone. Tears formed in my eyes. I got to school but classes had already started. I wanted to burst into tears. I couldn't walk in looking like this. I dived into the nearest toilet and looked at my face. It was a right state. My eyes were red and puffy, my skin blotchy, my hair lank and lifeless. I splashed water on my face and gulped some too. In my rush and panic to get to school I'd almost forgotten about my hunger. Now it returned with increased nausea.

After taking a few minutes to compose myself I walked to class. When friends asked I said I'd just slept in after staying up late. There was no way I could tell them the truth.

For the rest of that week Linda's attitude softened. We were still restricted to our room, still could only go to the toilet when she said but we were fed our meals, went to school on time and although there was a danger we might succumb to mind-numbing boredom there was not the constant fear of being hit or subjected to forms of punishment that would be outlawed in a prison. The reason for this soon became clear. Social services were paying a visit. The planned contact with my brother and sister wasn't going ahead, which I was desperately sad to hear, but Claire, my recently appointed social worker, wanted to check how things were going.

Watching Linda turn on the charm was sickening. She made it out like I had the best life with her.

'Of course, Jade has her moments and I'm required to discipline her but on the whole she's a good child.'

'Jade, how have things been with you?'

This was another chance to speak up. I didn't owe Linda anything. It's not like keeping quiet before had earned me any plus points in her eyes. If anything she was worse. Even if I'd wanted to she made it practically impossible. As before, she hovered around, always in earshot. And what was the point of telling Claire anything? I felt embarrassed even thinking about the things Linda made us do – the naked showering, having to lie in your urine-soaked clothes. Saying it out loud would only make it worse.

I just had to accept this was my life and adapt, in the same way I'd had to adapt to my mum's inability to look after us. I felt cheated, though. It had been an easy decision to make when social services asked where I wanted to live but this wasn't the life I'd been promised, either by Linda or the social workers. There was no happy home life, there was no regular contact with my mum or dad and now even the meetings with Jack and Ellen were drying up. Everything reinforced the view I'd formed as a young child, when interrogated by teachers, that you couldn't trust adults.

Once the social worker's visit was out of the way, Linda could give up her pretence to be nice and she resumed her vindictiveness. She shepherded us into the bedroom and ordered us to take up our positions on the floor, with only our notepads and Lego for amusement. I couldn't even bring myself to draw a picture. I just felt so hacked off. I was sitting with my back to the other girls when there was a flutter and a little paper note landed by my side. I looked round and caught Sara's eye but she turned away shyly as soon as she saw me. I unfolded the note.

'Can you show me how to draw like you do?' it said.

I looked around again. She turned her head too and this time when I caught her eye she smiled. I nodded and shuffled over to where she was. I drew a quick outline of a face and sketched out the eyes and nose, showing her how to get the alignment right. She then had a go. I stopped her before she made some basic errors – the eyes too high, too far apart, the mouth where the nose should be. We took a few goes but after half an hour she was picking it up.

'You're amazing,' she whispered when I added a few touches to bring the eyes out. I smiled, remembering how I felt when Mum showed me how to draw. It was like a magician revealing their tricks, like she'd given me a secret code to a new world that had previously been closed to me.

We were so engrossed I hadn't noticed Arlene had shuffled silently over to see what we were doing. Without speaking I motioned to the pad and gestured if she'd like me to show her. She nodded. I drew some eyes. I loved doing them and showed the tricks to get them right. I built up the face and drew in some hair, another thing people often get wrong. Arlene had a go and did very well. They both had a natural talent. I wondered if anyone had ever sat down with them and tried to nurture it before.

Another thing I've always had a knack for was love hearts. I could draw them perfectly. I showed them and they both nodded eagerly. They tried them but theirs were messy so I showed them how to do it a bit neater. They seemed impressed. Next I showed them better colouring technique as I'd seen some of the scribbling they'd done with felt tips and they were very untidy. They picked that up quickly too. Here we were, three outcasts brought together by the ill-treatment of our carer, bonding over some sketches, doing the one thing we had to amuse us.

We should have known it wouldn't last.

Huddled over our pads in the middle of the room we didn't hear the door open until the customary screech of the hardened paper.

'What are you doing?'

'Drawing, like you said we could,' I said.

'Not like that. I want you facing away – and not talking.'

'We weren't talking,' I said. 'We were drawing.'

'Don't be cheeky.'

'But I'm not, that's what we were doing. I swear.'

She split us up into our corners for the last hour before teatime. Trust Linda to spoil our fun. She thought she was punishing us by letting us draw in the pads. She was probably furious that we'd found a way to have fun. I was cursing the fact that every nice thing seemed to be frowned upon when another note landed by my side.

'Thanks,' it said, next to a smiley face.

Maybe out of the darkness of our situation there was a shaft of light. And maybe I wasn't as alone as I feared.

Chapter 16

I knew I was dead the moment the paper fell from the door. I'd been so careful. It had been weeks since Linda had last had to replace it. I'd become skilled at prising open the door without dislodging it. On the couple of times it had slipped out I'd been able to catch and slot it back into exactly the same position.

Now, as I looked down to where it lay on the carpet after tumbling from the doorframe, I knew I was in trouble.

'Oh hell,' Sara whispered when she saw my predicament.

I picked it up and examined it like an archaeologist might do a relic they'd just dug up, looking for a clue to where it fitted into the general picture. There was a groove but the folds had unravelled slightly so it had lost its shape. I tried squeezing it into where I'd thought it had fallen from and closed the door, but it didn't hold. It turned it, squashed it, tried to remould it but it was no use. The best I could hope for was to jam it in and wait for it to fall out when Linda next barged in. Then I'd be for it.

She'd get a new piece of toilet paper and we'd start all over again. It would be super squeaky for a while until I learned how to master it once more.

I had to hand it to her – it was a really effective alarm system. What I wondered, in the hours when I lay awake each night, was how did she discover it. Did she try other paper, cardboard, bits of plastic until she found the one that had the desired squeak? There were times when opening the door, with the paper wedged there, was suicide. It never ceased to amaze me how fast she could get up those stairs.

It wouldn't be long before she came back to check on us. I had a choice: get back to my position on the floor or make it to the bathroom, which was the reason for getting up anyway. I desperately needed a drink. After accusing me of talking last night I'd gone without breakfast and lunch but she'd softened her stance enough to give me a punishment tea biscuit and some ham.

I decided to go for it. If she was going to catch me anyway I might at least try to quench my thirst. I tiptoed out of the room and heard her talking. She was on the phone, no doubt to one of her children. I was probably good for a couple of minutes. I slipped along to the bathroom. Previous mistakes had taught me not to pull the flush if using the toilet and not to run water down the plughole. Now I put my mouth around the tap and poured the water directly in. It required nimble handwork so as not to choke yourself. The last thing you wanted was to cough your guts up in the bathroom and send her running. I glugged some water down my throat and headed back to the room. I could still hear her on the phone so there wasn't the same urgency to get back in position. I fiddled with the toilet paper and got it wedged the best I could.

Since the day I'd first taught them drawing we'd passed more notes to each other. It was better than risking getting caught talking, and also more fun. Sometimes Sara and I passed notes at Arlene's expense to wind her up. When I'd resumed my position she passed one to me.

'She's just old and mean.'

She was meaning her older sister, who'd been having a go at her. I giggled and reached for a pen to begin my reply.

The door screeched in alarm. I jumped out of my skin and dropped the note. I turned and saw the hardened toilet paper on the floor. Linda bent down and held it up like a trophy.

'Ah, who's been up to the toilet?'

'No one. It just fell now.'

'Liar! You know what happens to liars, Jade.'

I braced myself, trying to cover my legs as best I could. They were always her favourite targets when you were sitting on the floor. She strode forward but stopped. Something had caught her eye. It was the note. I tried to grab it but she was too fast. She slapped away my hand and unfurled it.

'Who wrote this?'

Sara cowered, burying her head in her knees. Arlene, who probably didn't know the content of the note, could tell enough by her reactions that this was serious.

'Who?'

I imagined the beating Sara would get once Linda found out. It was bad enough when you were in bed but to be hit on the floor was the worst. Sara would be kicked about like a rag doll.

'I did.'

'Jade!' Sara said, lifting her head.

'It's okay, Sara,' I whispered.

'I might have known it was you,' Linda sneered. 'Horrid child. After all I do for you.'

If I hadn't been so scared I might have laughed. I steeled myself for the blow I expected to come but Linda had other ideas. Pain shot through my skull as I was wrenched backwards by my hair. She yanked my hair again and slapped me hard across the side of my head, over the ear my mum had hit before. I scrambled to stop myself falling over completely, flailing at her arms to try to break her grasp. She pulled on my hair again. The pain was unbearable but then a kick to my thigh had me reaching to protect my legs. She hauled me over to the bed and for one terrifying second I feared she was going to smack my head on the frame. Instead she rammed me up against it.

'Think you're smart do you?'

'It was about Arlene,' I spluttered.

That stopped her momentarily in her tracks. It must have put some doubt in her mind because she read the note again and let go of my hair.

'Get back in your corner,' she said.

'What are you saying about me?' Arlene chipped in.

'You shut up!' Linda said. She had a funny look on her face, like she suspected she'd overreacted but couldn't be sure. After some huffing and puffing and shouting she stormed out of the room, returning moments later with a new piece of paper to jam the door shut.

When she'd gone, Arlene shot me a filthy look.

Great. Now I was going to get it from both sides. Arlene, I figured, we'd be able to explain it to but Linda was going to get her revenge for this. Arlene saw the funny side when she read the note and Sara was very thankful that I'd spared her a beating.

But sure enough, with Linda, we all had to suffer another few days of missed meals and much more frequent checks on us to make sure we were sitting in silence in our corners.

This must be what prison is like, I thought over those days, as another hour crawled by in the Bad

Room. In fact, I imagined prison would be better. I thought of the places where Mum was held. They got to see visitors, exercise and eat three meals a day. I remembered that one of the prisons had had a basketball net. Others had games rooms. It didn't seem too bad. At least in prison you knew your sentence. You could tick off the days until you got out. In the Bad Room we had no idea how long we'd serve.

The days had stretched into weeks and into months. The evenings got lighter and that made it worse. Being confined to our room when you could hear children playing outside was particularly torturous. In the winter months, although it was hell, we were enclosed in our own little world. When it was dark outside it was hard to imagine anyone else having fun. Now, though, hearing the excited chatter and laughter hammered home how much we were missing out.

Not a week had gone by without some kind of punishment from Linda. Invariably it was me who got it. However, I don't know if they were following my lead or they'd just had enough of life in the room, but Arlene and Sara began to be bolder. We were forging an alliance – and we'd need to if we were going to survive.

Chapter 17

It didn't matter what the circumstances were, it was always a risk taking that first look out of the room. The biggest fright came when you peered round the door and saw her standing there, right outside. Part of me still hadn't recovered from the first time that happened. Sometimes, if your timing was right, you could bluff it by saying something like, 'I thought I'd heard you call us for our tea.' If it was late – and by that I mean past the time when Linda expected us to be in bed – then you knew you were for it.

And so whenever I opened the door, if I achieved this without too much of a squeak from the hardened bit of paper, the next hazard was what waited outside.

What brought me to the door tonight was a desperate need to go to the toilet. I cursed myself for gulping too much water earlier. I should have known it would go right through me. I'd been sleeping and when I woke it was the first thing to hit me. The next was how light it still was. I hated that. I'd been in such a deep sleep I hoped it was morning. Seeing Arlene propped up awake in her bed and then hearing the noise from the street outside told me it was still relatively early. It was the start of summer. We'd be breaking up from school in a few weeks but the only thing to which we could look forward was that, with the arrival of the Ukrainian girls, Linda might treat us a bit nicer.

This evening Linda had a friend over so I felt a bit safer getting up and going to the toilet. She didn't normally make a scene when someone was in the house. Even though you could never be too careful.

I slowly peered around the door. *Oh my God.*

'You are not going to believe this,' I said, battling to keep my voice to a whisper.

'What?' they both said.

'Come and see this.'

Even by our standards we'd had quite a week of it. Endless persecution it seemed. I don't think any of us had made it through the day with three meals. I'd had to resort to swiping some muffins from a bake sale at school in order to have something to eat. I'd shared them with Sara on the way home. It had been that kind of week. So with that in mind they both needed further persuading. I motioned them forward eagerly. They must have known from my wide eyes that it was worth risking getting up for. Arlene rolled out of her bunk as

Sara dropped down from hers. After negotiating the creaky floorboards they joined me at the doorframe.

'Look what she's done,' I said, urging them to poke their heads around the door and look down the landing.

In between our room and the bathroom, spanning the floor of the hallway in a criss-cross pattern all the way to the toilet, were slats of wood. It took me a while to work out exactly what they were. Then I got it. They were the beams from the bunk bed in Lisa's room, most likely from the bed I used to sleep in, back when things were different. When I thought she was nice.

When had she done this? How had none of us heard?

It was like something you'd see in a film. They were so tightly woven it would be nearly impossible to get a foot between the gaps and lift it so as not to move them and make a sound. She'd blocked off the entire route to the toilet. That was obviously her plan. With her friend over she wouldn't be able to check on us quite so much. She probably suspected that, as she was occupied, we might chance something. And so she needed another deterrent.

'I don't believe it,' Arlene said. She shook her head, sighed and went back to bed. There was not a lot that shocked her but I suspected that even for her this was a new one.

'Sorry,' Sara said, shrugging. She too navigated her path safely back to her bunk.

I thought about joining them but then my bladder throbbed again. I had no choice.

'I've got to go,' I told them. 'I'm desperate.'

'You're crazy,' Arlene said.

'Good luck,' Sara added, biting her nails.

I stepped into the hall and took stock of this challenge. There were too many to jump. If I hit one of them it would make an almighty racket, plus I'd have to take a run up and even if I managed to clear them I'd have her up here like a shot. There was absolutely no route through without knocking them about.

Then I had an idea.

I put my back against one wall of the hall and hitched my feet up on the other side. They reached. I was effectively sitting, off the ground, across the hall. Painstakingly, I edged along the wall, terrified that at any moment my feet would slip and I would come crashing down on the beams. Then all hell would break loose. Then, it wouldn't matter that she had a guest visiting. She'd be up here in no time.

Inch by inch, I bumped and slid along the wall, like James Bond trying to evade laser beams in some arch villain's lair. I'm sure if I had stopped and seen myself it might have been quite funny, but when you're straddled across a hall, several inches off the floor, with a bladder fit to burst, all you can think about is making it to the other side.

To my own astonishment I cleared the last piece of wood and dropped down outside the toilet. Having relieved myself, I was careful not to pull the flush. Ever since Arlene pointed out the noise the water made down the pipes I'd not made that mistake again. After I was done I had a quick slug of water. Not too much. I didn't want to repeat this escapade. Then I had to do the same again and hitch and slide back along the hall-way. It was a bit easier now without the same pressure on my bladder.

I reached halfway when my body froze in fear. A door downstairs opened. Surely not. My heart was thumping so hard I could swear it was going to break free from my chest.

Who was it? Where were they going? Please God, not her. Not upstairs.

I heard a voice. It was her!

For a moment every instinct told me to abandon the mission, drop down and sprint for the room. Fear, though, kept me stuck to the wall.

She was talking to her friend while still standing in the doorway for what seemed like a lifetime. I lost all feeling in my legs. They could fall to the floor now and I wouldn't be able to do a thing to stop them.

Then she moved. My hands were so sweaty I might slide off. Surely she was going to be heading for the stairs. Then I realised with relief she was going into the kitchen. Thank goodness.

I shuffled along, cleared the beams of wood, made it into the room, gently closed the door and made sure the paper was in its right position.

'Well?' Sara whispered.

'Made it. Not easy!'

Arlene smiled. 'How?'

'Along the wall. I hitched up and shuffled along.'

They both fell into giggles, no doubt imagining what I'd looked like. I tiptoed across the floor, careful to avoid the creaks again and made it back into bed. What had seemed like mission impossible was now mission accomplished. I was buzzing and felt a huge sense of satisfaction.

'Remember,' I whispered to the others. 'We don't know those bits of wood are there.'

We could hear Linda say goodbye to her friend. There was the door closing and then the unmistakable clump, clump of her boots coming up the stairs. Even though there was no evidence I'd done anything wrong my heart still pounded when she approached. I slid further down the covers and pulled them up to eye level. There was a bit of noise outside the room. Was she moving the wood? It was hard to tell. I pulled the covers over my head.

I heard the squeak that signalled the door opening.

'Who's been up?'

My whole body throbbed so much I was sure she would tell my guilt through the bedclothes.

'Who has been in the toilet?'

Oh God. She knew. The unflushed pan. A give away.

Stay firm, girls, stay firm. If no one tells, she might think it was from earlier, when she'd lined us up for our humiliating showers. Maybe this was a trick to us to see if we would admit that we knew the beams were there.

I'll give her one thing. She was certainly committed to catching us out.

Don't fall for the trap, girls.

She was met with only silence.

We were learning. We were sticking together.

After what seemed like an age, she left. The door closed. Silence once again.

I let out a huge sigh into my pillow. I'd done it. It was a victory; a small one but I'd take it.

I lowered the sheets. I saw Arlene lying there staring at me.

'That was close.' The voice was Sara's above me.

Arlene put a finger to her lips and gestured to the door. She was right. We hadn't heard any more movement. Linda was probably right outside waiting to see if we gave the game away by talking.

I held my breath. I imagine they were doing the same too. No one wanted to miss even the tiniest sound. The noise from outside had died too. I could swear even the bird that until recently could still be heard chirping had fallen silent. It was like the world was holding its breath waiting to see what happened next.

Who would crack first?

I almost couldn't take it any longer. She was really keeping it going this time. Did she honestly think we'd start yakking just because she'd left the room? We'd been in here far too long to fall for that one.

Bang!

The door swung open so violently she must have kicked it.

My instinct was to duck under the covers but I couldn't take my eyes off her. She strode into the middle of the room.

'I'm going to ask this one more time. Who was in the toilet?'

She moved her eyes over all of us. I sat there, quilt to my nose, scared to blink in case it gave the game away.

'Very well then.'

She took two steps over to Arlene's bed, ripped back the cover and grabbed her arm.

'Get up!' She hauled the teenager off the bed with such force she nearly flew onto the floor. With Arlene sprawling on the floor, one leg still on the bed, she strode over to our bunk. I pulled the quilt tight to me. It wasn't me she was after though. Not yet.

Up she reached. I heard the sounds of a struggle. Sara was kicking with all her might. That was unusual for her. I saw the covers wrenched off. An arm appeared over the side of the bunk, then Sara's chest. Still she tried to resist but Linda was too strong. She pulled again and the younger sister fell headfirst to the floor, only able at the very last moment to put out her arms to stop her neck potentially breaking.

I cowered into the corner of my bunk.

'You!' Linda sneered and pulled at the covers. She smacked me twice on the leg and pulled at the top of the sheets. I gripped on but they were coming away. She pulled and I lifted off with them. Once she'd got them off she grabbed any limb she could get hold of, an arm and a leg, and dragged me to the floor.

'Now stand up, all of you.'

We all shuffled to our feet, hair dishevelled, faces bright red, everyone, including her, breathing heavily.

'Who did it?'

I put my hand up, panting too hard to speak.

Smack! She whacked me over the head.

'Get on the floor!'

I didn't need telling twice. I dropped into a foetal position.

'You two. Back to bed.' To me: 'You will sleep on the floor all night. But not like that. Sit up.'

I did as I was told, my head ringing from where she slapped me. I sat, hands around my knees.

'Move away from the bed.'

I shuffled over a bit towards the window.

'Right, there. I don't want you thinking you can lean against the bed.'

Arlene and Sara had climbed back into their beds.

'Next time, when I ask a question I expect an answer. As for you, Jade, I will be checking all night to make sure you don't move. Got it?'

I nodded but kept my head down.

Still breathing heavily, she finally left the room.

I hugged my legs closer, lay my head on my knees and tried to go back to sleep. I might have won a small victory but the battle was hers.

That was a big one. In the run-up to the end of term she sought to punish me any chance she got. For days she sent me to school with no lunch. One or two days I could cope with but when I had to go three days with only a meagre tea, a bowl of cereal and then nothing for lunch, it took its toll. My friend Leanne saw that I was desperate and brought in some extra food so I would at least have something to eat. I hated the thought of being treated like a charity case but I was so hungry I was grateful for her help and compassion.

Linda's cruelty knew no bounds. When the school held a mufti day and we could wear our casual clothes she forced Sara and me to wear our uniform. It sounds trivial but I felt acute embarrassment turning up in my usual skirt and blouse when everyone else used it as a chance to showcase their personal style. She might as well have dressed me in overalls that said 'Foster Kid' on the back. After a couple of days like this, when other kids picked on me for wearing my uniform, Leanne helped out by bringing in an additional top so I could change. That made my day, until someone, perhaps a teacher, mentioned it to Linda that I'd got my days confused. My punishment was two days without dinner.

Social services, I was sure, provided Linda with money so I could attend school trips, but that was a treat denied to me. Whenever I asked if I could go on a day trip to a museum or a sight of historical interest she refused. The same went for the trips to nearby theme parks. While my classmates excitedly left for the day I had to stay behind. It was yet another reminder that I was different. When it came to bigger trips, like those week-long cultural visits to Italy or Germany or a skiing adventure that some children went on, there was no way she allowed it. It was soul destroying. I felt like a second-class citizen. Almost worse than the beatings and feeling a prisoner in the Bad Room was the psychological torture of social exclusion. I felt like my sense of self was slowly being eroded away to nothing. Who was I anymore? Linda was chipping away every ounce of my confidence. I had been doing well at school and had enjoyed it but my results started to slip. It was hard to concentrate when all you were thinking about was when and where you might next find something to eat. I was regularly late for school in the morning because she hadn't woken me after keeping me up most of the night.

The only silver lining to the dark cloud that seemed to follow me around every day was that when I was forced to stay behind in school sometimes Sara had to do the same. Teachers put the two of us in the music room and left us to our own devices for the day. It was like the school equivalent of our situation at Linda's. Trapped in a room with just each other for company. At least at school we could talk and the bond between us grew stronger. We were able to formulate plans.

Linda continued to insist that we walk to school separately. We worked out that she could only see us as far as the first set of traffic lights. Before we reached them we walked on opposite sides of the road. Once we were past those we crossed over and chatted the rest of the way. At the end of the day we did the same in reverse so it looked as though we still weren't speaking. The more I got to know Sara and Arlene the more I realised that Linda had been mean to say all those awful things about them. They were just kids, they'd been in care for most of their lives and they didn't deserve to have her calling them horrible names. Even though she'd shoved us together in the same room she'd done everything she could think of to drive a wedge between us. Through our shared misery, though, we had bonded. It meant life in Linda's house was marginally more bearable.

By the time of my twelfth birthday Linda's behaviour had improved slightly. That's because she knew my social workers would be making contact. Social work passed on a gift from my mum but there was no other form of contact. My meetings with my siblings were few and far between. Staff shortages or Linda claiming she was ill meant these sessions often got cancelled at short notice. During the summer holidays Linda had the girls from Ukraine staying so she relaxed her rules temporarily. When Terry was off work we went on the odd day trip to Blackpool and their family would come round to visit, so we would be wheeled out and have to pretend that we loved life there. The reality, however, was that it was interminably dull over those long summer weeks. Still not allowed out, I never saw any friends for the entire time and it was cruel to have to go bed early when it seemed like the whole neighbourhood was having a party outside. I longed to get back to school because, although I also suffered there – through lack of food, not having new clothes and not being able to take part in trips and other activities – my friends were my escape. That's where I laughed, where I was happy, where I was able to be a bit of a child and I felt free. Even stepping out the house in the morning I would fill my lungs, stare up at the sky and just feel alive, if only for a few minutes. At school, I could give myself a pep talk: 'This will get better – you've got this.' I could escape my miserable thoughts and at lunch club we were allowed on the computers so I could listen to music, if only for a few brief minutes. Being able to step outside of that house for seven hours a day recharged my strength so that I could put up with whatever was going to be thrown at me once I returned. But during the summer holidays, I was trapped. There was no recharge button. I felt suffocated.

As soon as the Chernobyl girls left and school resumed, however, the battle of wits began again.

The wooden beams in the hallway had not made a reappearance but since I'd been caught that night I'd avoided detection after Arlene passed on her tip.

'Use the bidet instead of the toilet,' she said. 'You don't need to flush and it's not as obvious.'

It was simple advice but it seemed to work. Perhaps inspired by my efforts to defy Linda, the girls grew a little braver in going to the toilet, even though they'd been told not to.

The nights were growing darker again and sometimes there would be no light upstairs when we were making our way silently to the bathroom. One evening we all managed to get there and back without being detected. Or so we thought. It was late when Linda stormed into the room with a triumphant look on her face.

'Who has been up when they weren't supposed to be?'

'We haven't left the room,' I said. 'We've been here the whole time.'

'None of us have been,' Arlene added.

'Get up all of you.' She stood there, arms crossed, tapping her foot while we crawled out of bed. 'Then how do you explain this?' she said, leading us to the door and into the hallway where she switched on the light.

Only now did we see that the whole floor had been sprinkled with white.

'That's talcum powder,' she said, a weird smile on her face.

My stomach lurched. There, over to the sides of the carpet – where we'd avoided the squeakiest of floorboards – were what looked like three sets of footprints leading up to and back from the bathroom. Busted!

We all had to spend hours sitting up as punishment, making me late once more for school the next day. During those long dark hours when you had nothing to do but sit there I almost wished she'd hit us. Sometimes being beaten was preferable. It was over quicker and if you were in bed at the time she unleashed her fury you could at least try to protect yourself with the duvet. There were times, though, when sitting shivering in a nighties now three sizes too small a freezing cold night was welcome – those times were preferable to her kicking you so hard with her black leather boots that you felt your leg was broken, or your insides were bleeding, if she caught you in the stomach. And if she caught you in the back, like she did once to Sara and me, it meant sitting on the floor was absolute agony. There was no position in which you could remotely find comfort. Then it was just a long night of misery that you spent praying for some kind of salvation. But there was none. It wasn't like anyone was coming for us or anyone was properly checking on us. We were on our own in the Bad Room. And it was only going to get worse.

Chapter 18

Living in such an oppressive situation meant the urge to rebel was sometimes too strong to resist.

Sara and I didn't mean to get into trouble when we left for school one winter morning, but we were passing the shop at the back of the building when we spied a bottle lying on the ground. It was an unopened bottle of Lambrini fizzy wine. We knew we shouldn't take it. Neither of us had tasted alcohol before and we were completely naïve to what it did to you. We just thought it would be cool to take it into school and tell our friends. Sara took possession of it and at break time she found me and said we should go to the toilets. Some of my friends and I went with her and we all crammed into a cubicle. We dared each other to have a sip but none of us had done so when a teacher walked in. It was Mr Johnston, our head of year teacher. He'd been told there were a lot of us up to no good. One of the girls rolled the bottle under another cubicle but it must have been obvious what we were doing. He found the wine and marched us all to his office. All I could think about was the trouble I'd get into when I got back to Linda's.

'Please don't tell Mrs Black,' I pleaded. 'She'll kill us.'

It was inevitable that the school would inform our foster carer and it was equally predictable that she would punish us.

'How dare you bring shame on me like that,' she said, sending us to the Bad Room.

We weren't allowed even the notepads or Lego that evening and we had to go another night without food or water. She also kept us late in the morning so we got in more trouble at school for that. I had to accept the wine incident was my own fault but I felt that slowly a picture was forming in the school that I might be a problem child.

'How did she ever become a foster carer?' I asked Sara on the way to school one day. 'She's so mean. It's as though she hates children, yet she's got so many of her own, takes in foster children and the ones from Chernobyl.'

'I think she had a neighbour who had children and when that lady was rushed to hospital one day social services asked Linda if she could step in and look after them,' Sara said. 'She did and the social workers thought she did such a good job they asked her about taking more children in on a longer-term basis.'

'I can just imagine her turning on the charm,' I said.

'She used to say things to us about stuff that a family member used to do to her. Abuse and stuff. It was horrible,' Sara said.

She went on to describe a little of what Linda had told them – that she had suffered a miserable time as a child. It seemed incredible to think that, if she'd not had a happy childhood, why she'd want to put other kids through that. I began to wonder if she'd ever been properly assessed and whether, if she were, social services would still think she should be allowed to look after children.

It was also remarkable to think that Terry had no idea any of this was going on. All the time he must just have thought we were kids being kids, playing upstairs. On Saturdays we sometimes still went into town with them both and played happy families as though nothing was ever wrong. It wasn't like we could speak to him about his wife. That just wasn't an option. Similarly, we wouldn't dream of saying anything to any of their children. Whenever they came round to visit it was one of the few times we were allowed downstairs to eat normally. It was a wonder we still knew how to sit at a table and use a knife and fork, we were so used to having our dinner on our knees and our evening meal being no more than two biscuits and a slice of ham.

Another Christmas came and went and Linda performed the same trick as she'd done the year before.

We were allowed to open what presents we had but come 2 January she removed them and stored them in her dining room. A new year it might be but it felt her only resolution was to come up with new ways to humiliate us.

Although she had female children of her own, she was completely unsympathetic to the sensitivities of adolescent girls. I felt particularly sorry for Arlene, whose body was developing. At a time when her privacy should be respected she was forced to shower in front of us and endure Linda making comments about her body shape and hair growth. It was disgusting but it wasn't long before I found out first hand how insensitive she could be to women's issues.

On the day I got my period I was crying my eyes out. I thought I was dying. I only noticed when I woke up and was getting ready for school. She just handed me some Tampax and shouted instructions at me. She forced all three of us to wear them at bedtime so we wouldn't make more mess than we had to. I didn't know such things as sanitary towels existed. I felt unclean and ashamed. Luckily I had friends I could confide in who were more sympathetic, but in the house it was yet another thing to feel uncomfortable about. Even with her preferred sanitary method, there were bound to be accidents, yet Linda found a way to humiliate us with our laundry.

Her normal system was to put our dirty uniforms into the laundry basket on a Friday night to be washed over the weekend and returned to us clean for Monday morning. We were to bring it down to be washed but only when she called us. If she wanted to punish us, however, the call would never come. If we asked on a Saturday morning whether our clothes could be washed she blamed us.

'It's your fault your clothes won't be clean,' she said.

'But you never called us,' I complained.

She grabbed the dirty washing out of the basket, sorted it out into our bundles and threw them on the floor.

'Each of you pick up your dirty clothes, put them under your pillow. Tonight you will all sleep with them. This is what you get for not bringing them to me. Maybe then you will remember to bring them down at the right time in future.'

We had no choice but to do what she said.

On Monday morning it was horrible putting on clothes you knew were dirty from the previous week. Linda only gave us three blouses and two skirts so already, on a good week, we were making them last, but if that wasn't bad enough sometimes she refused to give us clean socks, forcing us to wear the same pair over and over again. This from the woman who'd told me when I first arrived how important it was not to give kids a reason to bully me. Now, nearly two years on, she was hell bent on giving them every reason. It was like she wanted me to be known as a gypsy or poor kid.

One Friday morning it got too much. I refused to put on the same pair of dirty socks I'd worn all week.

'I'm not going to school!' I shouted, my face burning up and the tears filling my eyes.

'Stay off and you'll get into even more trouble. They're already on to you at that school,' she said and slapped me hard across the head.

Normally that would have been my cue to shut my mouth and leave for school crying, but that day I felt she was pushing me too far.

'I'll go to school,' I said, through my tears. 'And I'll tell them why I was refusing to come in.'

For a brief moment I could have sworn a frightened look came over her face, as though she was working out the implications. She was always confident that we would never tell on her. Maybe now she wasn't so sure.

By the time I got to school I thought better of it. As before, I felt I wouldn't be believed and the consequences of speaking out would be serious. It just became yet another morning when I turned up late with swollen bloodshot eyes. I skipped first period to compose myself before facing classmates who didn't need a new reason to laugh at me because I was the tragic foster kid.

And they had plenty of opportunities to laugh at me.

Like every child that age we were at the mercy of every bug that went around school; not just colds and flu but also head lice. Once one person got it in class soon everyone would have it.

When, inevitably, nits came to our house, it was Sara who got them first. Linda might have been able to prevent them spreading but she refused to buy us the special shampoo that helped eradicate them, so within a week or so we were all riddled with them.

The eggs showed up most clearly on my hair as it was long, dark and went down my back.

'Let me cut them out,' Linda said, when they were so obvious it was disgusting. 'I used to be a hairdresser. I know what I'm doing.'

She marched us all into the bathroom naked and got out her scissors. They weren't like proper hairdresser scissors, they were ones she kept in the kitchen to cut the meat, but they might as well have been garden shears for the job they did on my locks. She hacked off so much it resembled the mullet Kat Slater used to sport on *EastEnders*. Linda's daughter Rebecca was a hairdresser and when she came round and saw me she said, 'Who's cut Jade's hair?'

'Me,' Linda said.

Rebecca's face told its own story. She was horrified. I was traumatised.

I didn't want to go to school the next day but Linda forced me to. Not only was my hair hacked to bits but she'd finally bought the head lice shampoo and it stank. Everyone would know I had nits. My friends were so upset on my behalf when they saw me. They could tell immediately it had been hacked at. Leanne had just been given straighteners so the next day she brought them in to try to help me. It helped me look a little more respectable but when I got home Linda pounced on me.

'Who's been touching your hair? You look like a slag.'

I was getting called names at school for having nits and at home the torment was never ending. As punishment for 'tarting' myself up she refused to give me dinner that night.

I couldn't wait for breakfast the following morning but when I went downstairs she'd left nothing, no cereal and no packed lunch, for me.

By the time I got to school I was desperately hungry. I'd had no opportunity to tell my friends so no one had any extra food or money that I could have. The school was organising a collection for something and I spied some cash lying in a tray. One pound would buy me a sandwich. I didn't want to steal but I was at my wits' end. I just needed to eat something. When I thought no one was looking I slipped a pound into my pocket. As soon as I did it I felt bad – and I felt even worse when a hand appeared on my shoulder. It was my new head of year teacher, Miss Ashton. She took me to my office and sat me down.

'Are you having problems at home?'

I wanted to cry and tell her everything. This could be the chance to bring an end to Linda's cruelty. I just needed to put my faith in the school and the system. Yet somehow the words wouldn't come. Instead a voice in the back of my head said, 'Don't trust them. It will only make it worse.'

'No,' I said firmly.

There was a long pause while she looked at me. It was as if she was willing me to have a rethink and tell her. She had a kind face and on some level I suspected she meant well but I had had years of conditioning. I wouldn't tell.

'Can I give you some advice?' she said. 'Whenever you feel like stealing try to think of the feeling like a big blue monster, like the one out of the movie *Monsters Inc*. Think of that compulsion like a monster and chase it out of your mind.'

To her I must have just looked like another naughty rebelling child, when the truth was I had no faith in my school to help me. As far as I was concerned they were in league with Linda and the social workers. They kept me in misery, denied me basic freedoms and, apart from the odd isolated contact meeting every few months, blocked me from seeing the brother and sister I loved or from receiving any updates, if there were any, on my mum and dad.

Growing increasingly resentful, I began pushing back against Linda. When she told me off I answered back, when she tried to hit me I resisted. I'd watched Arlene and how she sometimes lost the plot with Linda. For the most part she remained a quiet girl but when she flipped she went psycho and I could see Linda was scared of what she was capable of. By now Arlene was 15 and towering over Linda. She was also experiencing problems at school and we would hear reports coming back of her trying to run away from her class and locking herself in cupboards. She could be a real handful when she wanted to be. As it was with Sara and me, all of Arlene's problems could be traced back to her foster home. Through tears of anger, she told us she had tried to tell her teachers what was going on but no one believed her. Everything was brushed under the carpet.

As well as watching how Arlene fought with Linda, I saw how our foster carer responded to what she saw as insolent behaviour. For two days after one of their blazing rows Arlene was sick. She threw up her breakfast and was off her food for the rest of the day.

The following morning our cereal was lined up as usual but Linda, as I remembered she'd done the previous morning, was keen to point out to Sara and me which ones were ours and which was Arlene's. For another day Arlene was sick.

'My breakfast tastes horrible,' she said on the third morning, when Linda had specified again which bowl she was to use. 'I think she's putting salt or something in my cereal.'

No way, we thought, could she be serious? Would Linda really stoop so low to effectively try to poison a child?

'Remember when we were on holiday,' Sara said, referring to the last trip all of us made to the caravan park, 'when she was mad with Terry.'

I did remember. We'd all been horrified when, after Linda and Terry had argued about something, she spat in his scrambled eggs before serving them to him. If she could do that to her own husband there was no telling what she'd do to us.

We all started sniffing our food and tasting little bits at a time.

Arlene went to school and must have told someone her suspicions because later that day a call came into the house from a teacher asking Linda about the allegation.

'That's preposterous,' we heard Linda say. 'If it happened it's more likely her sister or Jade who did it. You know what kids are like.'

Despite the threat that she might poison my food, I couldn't help but try to push back when she turned particularly nasty with me. She never showed the same fear as she did with Arlene, though. She just stepped up the brutality.

One night, when she tried to get me out of bed to make me sit on the floor, she grabbed me by the hair and pulled as hard as she could. Not only did she haul me to the floor but it felt like she had ripped the hair from my head. Sure enough, when I looked up she was standing staring at a clump of dark hair in her hand.

'See?' she screamed, dropping the hair on the floor. 'That's what happens when you don't just do as you're told!' She stormed out of the room and slammed the door shut.

Nursing my throbbing scalp I crawled over and collected my strands of hair. Miss Ashton had said something about telling them should anything happen in future they should know about. Now was the time to test that.

In the morning I went to school and sought out the deputy head, Mr Smith. I handed him the clump of hair Linda had ripped out and told him what had happened.

'Do you want to report your foster carer?' he said. 'I can't notify social services without your consent.'

It felt like that first incident year ago when Linda slapped me and my mum reported it. Then I'd felt social services didn't take it seriously. I imagined the meeting that would take place, where I'd have to tell on Linda while she listened to my every word. Then I imagined how brutal her punishment would be once we were alone.

'I don't know,' I said. 'I don't think so. Not at the moment.'

I left his office feeling more broken and alone than I had ever felt before. I wasn't even sure what I wanted him to say – that I never needed to go back there, that the school would deal with Linda so that she'd never hit or punish me again?

I only knew one thing. If my school and social services were unable to help – then I had to take matters into my own hands.

Chapter 19

'Come on, girls, hurry up.'

Our PE teacher Miss Roberts was always on our case to get changed as quickly as possible. There was always pandemonium while we all changed into our t-shirts and tiny shorts. As soon as we were ready we began to file out into the hall.

'Jade,' Miss Roberts said. 'Hang back.'

Not wanting to do anything that split me from my friends, I protested but she was insistent. When everyone else had left the changing room she looked down at my legs. 'What happened to you?'

I followed her gaze to the bruises clearly visible on both thighs – reminders of when Linda had whacked me the night before for daring to go to the toilet for a drink of water. Suddenly put on the spot I felt incredibly self-conscious. I just wanted to get out there and play whatever sport we were going to do that day with my pals. The last thing I wanted was an interrogation.

'Oh, those. It's nothing. A girl I live with, Sara, and me were messing about. It looks worse than it is. Can I go now?'

'Are you sure?' Miss Roberts said, frowning, 'they don't look like nothing to me.'

'Yeah, honestly. It was just from a play fight.'

She let me go and I raced outside, hoping no one saw me being kept back. The last thing I wanted was any more reasons for people to think there was something up with me. I didn't think about it again for the rest of the school day. It was a Friday and I trudged home, heart heavy at the prospect of another weekend to endure. Returning home to Linda's I stepped through the door to find her standing there waiting for me.

Slap!

Without saying a word she whacked me around the head. I recoiled and put up my hands but she slapped me again. Then again.

'Ow! What are you doing? What have I done?'

I tried to move out of the way but she had me cornered. Again she hit me but I managed to block it.

'What have you been saying about me?'

Only then did I manage to look into her manic blue eyes and flushed face.

'What are you on about? I haven't said anything.'

'Why did your teacher call me to ask about some bruises you had?'

Now I got it. Miss Roberts must have called or spoken to someone who decided to check it out.

'It was only my PE teacher,' I said, still cowering behind my arms in case of further blows. 'She saw them when I was changing. I told her Sara did it. Honest. I didn't tell her anything.'

She held up her hand as though about to strike. I jerked back in anticipation.

'I don't believe you. Get to your room. Go straight to bed. Ungrateful brat. After all I do for you.'

I didn't need a second telling. I raced up the stairs, my ears ringing with more insults.

When the calls came later for Arlene and Sara to collect their trays I knew mine would not be there. As an extra punishment Linda had cooked a full dinner, making me suffer by having to lie there in bed watching them eat a plate of fish and chips.

The following morning was the same. No breakfast. Linda told me to stay in bed. I wasn't to get dressed. I just had to lie there. There was no lunch for me either, although Sara smuggled me some of her sandwich.

My stomach was in knots. The only thing I could do to alleviate the hunger pangs was sneak to the bathroom for gulps of water.

Come Sunday, Linda was still mad with me. For a second day I went without food, save for the scraps my roommates managed to save for me. I felt my spirit wilting. Even if I had been allowed to do anything I had no energy. All I wanted to do was lie in bed, curled up in a ball to try to stop the nauseous feeling.

When Monday morning came I was relieved to see a breakfast bowl there for me. I sniffed the cereal she left, just in case she'd thought of punishing me further.

'This is it,' I said to Sara on the way to school. 'I can't take any more of this. I'm going to run away.'

'Then I'm coming too.'

'No, Sara, you don't have to. It's not as bad for you. She hates me.'

'She hates us all,' Sara said. 'I want to come. I hate it there.'

And so we hatched a plan. Our only chance of escaping was while we were out of the house, on our way back from school. Sara managed to steal a couple of pounds so we could buy snacks for our journey. Once we had that we knew we were ready. I'd never felt excitement like it – nervous, scary excitement. I had such butterflies in my stomach but I knew I couldn't back out. This was our chance. So, two days later, when we'd worked up enough courage, we met up after school and instead of walking to Linda's we headed off on our own.

My suggestion was to head to the town where I used to live, seven miles away. I had no idea what we'd do there but it was the nearest place I knew and I just wanted to put some distance between us and Linda.

At least it was April and the weather was quite mild. It was thrilling to be out on our own. I felt the first sense of freedom I'd had in years. We chatted excitedly about all the things we wanted to do, as if this was the start of a big adventure. No one really gave us a second glance when we walked through the streets but once we got onto the country road a few drivers gave us funny looks.

We hadn't got far when a man on a bike stopped and spoke to us. He was an off-duty policeman and he asked what we were doing walking on a country road. We told him we were running away because our carer wasn't feeding us and sent us to bed early. He took us back to the house where he said he would sort it all out.

Linda flashed a look of disgust at us when he explained why he was with us, then she turned on the charm to the policeman.

'They were misbehaving so I grounded them. And now they're making up stories because they're mad at me,' she said.

We must have looked like a pair of petulant kids. Linda was all smiles as she said she'd make sure it didn't happen again. Then, once the door was closed, she had a go at us for embarrassing her and causing needless worry. Nothing changed. She just carried on as though nothing had happened. For the next few weeks it was the same cycle of being deprived of meals and forced to sit for hours, not moving. We needed to try something else and Sara suggested that we could stay with a friend of hers for a few days.

After school one Friday I met up with Sara and her friend Grace. She took us back to her house, where we told her mum about some of the treatment we endured. We told her about the set-up regarding our meals, the times Linda starved us and what life was like in the Bad Room. Grace's mum was shocked. We hadn't even told her about sleeping naked on the floor or being lined up for showers with no clothes on. Some things were still too embarrassing to talk about. She said we could stay for a couple of nights until she spoke to the school and social services. She phoned Linda to let her know we were safe. We listened in and could hear her put to Linda what we'd told her about her life there. From what we could hear, and from what Grace's mum told us when she came off the phone, Linda repeated her stance that we were just upset at being disciplined. For us, though, it didn't matter. Those two days were bliss. Sara and I were able to watch television, go outside and go to the toilet when we needed and not when someone told us we could. We ate proper hot meals and were treated with respect, not like tearaways who needed to be strictly controlled all the time.

I dreamt that I could live somewhere like this forever. But when Grace's mum spoke to the school and the teachers called Linda she turned on her kindly foster mother act. She said we were rebelling because when we'd been naughty she'd sent us to bed early. She told the school she would change and, if we behaved, we'd be able to stay up a bit later. We could go on school trips and she'd allow it if we wanted a bit more freedom to see our friends.

Social services told Grace's mum we had to go back to Linda's because there was nowhere else they could put us. They promised to monitor our situation and review it.

Once we were back in the house Linda did soften her stance a little. My social worker Claire came round to interview me but before her visit Linda sat me down and said, 'If you are very good and don't keep saying all these bad things about me you'll get to watch TV and you can go out with your friends.'

That would motivate any child. It was all I wanted, so I did as she asked and played down the worst of it. For a week or so she wasn't quite as strict but after that, once I imagined that she realised nothing was going to be done about her, she returned to her old ways. The promises over the trips were empty words. We never did get to hang out with friends. She was just saying what the school and social services wanted to hear.

I just thought, what's the point? It wasn't worth speaking out because when you did you weren't believed. Nothing would happen unless social services felt there was an issue and Linda seemed to have them wrapped around her finger. My teachers and social workers had formed a view of me that I just played up to get attention.

Both the school and social services warned me against running away. I pledged not to do it again and, in any event, Linda always kept the doors locked so there was no chance to get away once you were inside the house. Or so I thought.

One day when I came from school she was in her usual foul mood. Although she'd said she would be more lenient and not shut us away from the moment we came home from school, today she ordered me straight upstairs. I protested and she followed me up. She ordered me to sit in the corner and when I refused she hit me across the head.

'Don't disobey me,' she said, before storming out of the room and heading back downstairs.

I couldn't stand being under the same roof as her, so as soon as I thought it was safe, I snuck outside the room. I could hear Linda speaking in the kitchen. I could see the living-room door was shut. The front door was straight across from the bottom of the stairs – you could see it from the top of the stairs. That's when I saw them – the silver keys dangling in the lock. The keys were *never* in the door, as Linda and her husband mostly used the back door. This was an opportunity. It was now or never. I could hear her voice. She was still in the kitchen. I skipped down the stairs, holding on to the banister and making sure I didn't step on the noisy treads. I grabbed my shoes and approached the door. My hands fumbled with the keys; if she heard them jangling and came out, I was dead. Carefully I turned them in the lock, slowly opened the door and as soon as there was a big enough gap I ran out, not even stopping to shut it behind me.

Once I was outside I didn't know what to do. It wasn't like I had a plan, I just knew I had to run. So that's what I did. I ran until my lungs felt like they would burst outside my rib cage. It hurt to breathe. I headed towards the town centre, which was about an hour's walk away but tonight seemed to take me no time to reach. Eventually I stopped running and tried to get my breath back. I kicked around the streets for a bit, but at around 7 p.m. the police stopped me. Linda must have reported me missing or maybe they were suspicious about a girl my age wandering about on my own. They asked what I was doing. I told them I couldn't go back home; that my foster carer was horrible. They took me back home. Linda had visitors so she was keen to play the incident down as quickly as she could. Once again she told the police what they wanted to hear; it was all about how unruly I was and how I reacted when she tried to be strict.

It didn't matter what I tried to do, everyone just kept returning me to Linda's. Eventually I confided in my friend Leanne what was really going on in the house. I told her how Linda hit me and about the times she made me lie naked in the cold at night, or didn't wash our clothes. I felt ashamed telling her. She was horrified and upset on my behalf that I'd had to endure such treatment.

'Come to my house,' she said. 'We'll look after you. No one should have to live like that.'

We went back to her house and she told her mum everything I'd said about Linda. What I didn't know was that Leanne's mum worked for social services, so she reported Linda and called the police. Finally, it looked like action was being taken. Surely now Linda would have to answer for her cruelty? I couldn't believe it when the officer said they needed to return me to Linda. It was for social services to sort out with her. It was like Groundhog Day. It didn't matter who levelled what allegations against Linda, she seemed immune from censure. It was all so reminiscent of the early days when my mum complained. Social workers were just not interested. They only believed Linda when she said how difficult I was being.

She made the usual comments about how things would change then, once it had all blown over, she continued where she left off.

I was now into my fourth year in her house and it felt like I was serving a life sentence. Physically, I felt battered and bruised, and mentally I was in a downward spiral. There seemed to be no respite from this misery – which only presented itself in even more disturbing ways.

Chapter 20

What was even more remarkable about the situation with Linda was that, during our bleakest time in her house, social services placed another girl with her.

Megan was ten, nearly four years younger than me, and was a sweet child with a lovely bubbly nature. When she first arrived I felt like I was looking back in time. Linda couldn't have been nicer to her, playing the role of kindly granny. She put Megan in with Lisa, who was now in her early twenties but still very childlike at heart. I listened through the wall as Megan happily played on Lisa's games consoles and watched television.

Linda gave Megan the same spiel she had given to me – except now I was one of the bad girls who needed strict discipline.

'Stay away from them as much as you can,' she said. 'They're always getting into trouble, causing no end of issues with their schools. You don't want to end up like them.'

Yet unlike I had been with Arlene and Sara, Megan just wanted to play. She was intrigued by us older girls and naturally gravitated towards Sara and me, who were closest to her in age. She kept wandering through to our room. Linda, who was careful not to scold us in front of Megan – especially in those first few weeks – came in and tried to gently shoo her out.

Of course, during this period, social services were paying close attention and were keen to see how Megan would settle. Linda was on her best behaviour. I thought back to those early days, when life in this house had promised so much and was such a contrast to the years I'd spent with Mum and Paul. I thought of the times when Arlene had said to me that this was how they were treated. She had repeatedly warned me that one day it would turn. I never believed her. I thought I was different, someone special. Linda would never treat me the same. How naïve I was. Now I looked at Megan and I thought, please, no. Don't do this to her. Surely she would have a better outcome?

Megan's arrival, in early summer, meant the house was full and there was no visit from the children from Ukraine that year. We all had to adapt to the new girl's presence. Right from the start Linda insisted that she had to join in the humiliating night-time shower routine. By now Arlene was nearly 17 and looked a full-grown woman. She should have been granted some privacy but Linda continued to force her to queue up with the rest of us, mocking her with cruel comments about her body. Like any girl that age she was sprouting hair in places she probably never thought possible but Linda refused to let her shave. She and Linda locked horns regularly and when they kicked off it was explosive.

Little Megan was only witness to some of the spats and it never seemed to bother her. I just prayed she never got put in our room. None of us deserved it but she was so much younger and cheerier, so I hated to think of her cowering in fear if she ever had to witness Linda on the warpath.

Hopefully that would all be in the future, if at all. Maybe, I thought, with social workers keeping a close eye on the situation, Megan's arrival might be a good thing. It would force Linda to calm down. Maybe we'd all benefit.

For a few weeks and months, that's what it was like. Megan had the freedom of the house. She got to stay downstairs after her tea or come upstairs and play in Lisa's room. After a few minutes she'd breeze into our room. I'm sure she must have thought, like I did, that it was a strange set-up. Why were three teenagers spending all their time in there? Why did they eat all their meals in the room? Why did so little noise come from it?

But while I recalled wanting to get out of the room as quickly as I could when I was that age, Megan seemed to be increasingly intrigued. Sara and I humoured her and we played together. I drew pictures with her and taught her the same art techniques I'd shown the others. This only served to form a bond between us, so she wanted to come in even more. It meant Linda couldn't be as strict with us, but sometimes she couldn't help herself and ordered Megan away while she told us to go to bed or forced us to sit in our corners.

'You stay downstairs. Those girls have been very naughty and need to be disciplined,' Linda told her, sending her out.

Megan was wiser than her years and very quickly sussed out that the way Linda treated us wasn't right. She couldn't understand why there were nights when we weren't being fed at all. And we used that to our advantage.

'Do us a favour and bring us some food up,' I asked her when Linda had once again made us go without our dinner. 'Don't let Lisa know, though, or she'll tell on us.' Loving being given a secret task, Megan discreetly brought up some crisps or biscuits. She was careful not to let Lisa see what she was doing. I felt a little bad taking advantage of her but she loved helping us.

'Can I go into their room?' Megan asked Linda repeatedly. 'I want to sleep in the bunk above Arlene.' When I heard this I wanted to scream, 'No!'

To my relief Linda said the same. I suspected she was simply gauging how far she could push things with her new charge and was probably mindful of closer social-work monitoring. How long would it be before she turned? I remembered I got the best part of a year before she turned tyrannical. Would Megan get that long?

Although she had to stay with Lisa, as the weeks went on she spent even more time in with us. We always tried to encourage her to leave the Bad Room, but it seemed the more we pushed her away the more she wanted to be with us.

She kept on at Linda. I wanted to say to her, 'You don't know what it's like in here. You'll live to regret it.' On some level, though, I hoped it would never be so bad for her.

And so I wasn't able to put her off. Social services had notably reduced the frequency of their visits. Linda had to make less of an effort. I could sense a change coming. Sure enough, the next time Megan begged to be allowed into our room, Linda said, 'Okay, then. Take the bunk above Arlene. You can stay in with them from now on.'

Megan's fate was sealed. Linda didn't even afford her the luxury she had me of still having her dinners down-stairs. Immediately her plate was left at the bottom of the stairs. Megan was delighted. She felt like she was one of the gang, like she'd joined the cool club. If only you knew, I said to myself.

For the first few nights Linda wasn't quite as strict. She didn't check up on us as regularly. Maybe Megan being here might just be a good thing. Maybe Linda had grown tired of fighting with us. Perhaps the calls from the school, the report from Leanne's mum, the police bringing me home had all made a difference.

That was what I hoped. Experience should have told me otherwise.

Megan's presence in the room was in some ways a breath of fresh air. She always wanted to talk or play or ask questions. In any normal environment she would have been a joy to have around. In the Bad Room she was a lightning rod for Linda's short fuse.

'Ssh, Megan,' I said one night when she continued to talk after Linda had told us to go to sleep. 'If she has to come back in here she'll be cross.'

'We're only talking,' Megan said.

'I know but she says it keeps Terry awake.' Part of me couldn't believe I was repeating Linda's excuses for her, but when you're told something night after night it gets into your brain.

She shut up for a bit but I could tell she was restless and in no mood to go to sleep. I had no idea what time it was. When the nights were light the evenings seemed to go on forever, especially when you had nothing to do but lie there.

I had tried to warn Megan that Linda wasn't always the nice old lady she saw. Sounding just like Arlene and

Sara when they'd tried to tell me what she was like, I advised her she didn't want to get in her bad books. But just like me when I'd been in her position, she wouldn't listen. Now, rather than settling down, she tossed about in her bed.

'Don't be boring. Come on you, why are you not speaking?' Megan leaned over her bunk to peer down at Arlene, who was having none of it. 'Jade … Sara?'

'Megan, seriously, go to sleep. You'll get us all into trouble,' I said, now aware I was being even louder in an effort to quieten her.

'She's not that bad … I think you're just making up all that stuff …'

Megan never finished her sentence. The door swung open and there was Linda with a face like thunder.

'I thought I told you all to keep quiet in here.'

Instinctively, Sara, Arlene and I curled up in a futile attempt to make it look like we'd been sleeping all along. I peeked across at the other bunk to see Megan sitting upright. Guilty as charged.

'Megan! Are you keeping the others awake?'

'Sorry!' she said, looking startled at the sudden intrusion.

'Now you're in this room, Megan, you need to follow certain rules,' Linda said softly. 'The other girls know they have to be quiet so they don't keep Terry awake all night. He has to be up really early in the morning and needs his sleep. It's not fair if he keeps being disturbed now, is it?'

Megan shook her head and dropped back onto her pillow. She's lucky, I thought, that Linda's going easy on her. How long will that last?

'Now, no more talking, okay?'

She gave us all a withering look but retreated to the door and left us in milky darkness. For a few minutes all was quiet. She's obviously got through to Megan, I thought. Then I heard her stirring. I looked over. She was back sitting upright. I was going to tell her to try to get to sleep but I suspected Linda would still be outside the door. I gestured with my arm for her to get down. She did the opposite. Kicking back the covers she swung her legs over the side of the bed.

'What?' she said.

'Sssh!'

'What are you shushing for? She's gone. Don't be boring.'

I shook my head and pointed to the door. As Megan turned it opened so wide and sudden that it pinged back on its hinges.

'Megan! I told you to be quiet.'

The young girl had already dived back down and was scrambling to get under the covers. Linda was over in a flash and wrenched the duvet from her.

'I'm sorry. Can't sleep. I'm too hot.'

'Is that a fact? Right, then, get up.'

Megan continued to fight for the duvet and, eventually giving up, curled herself into a ball.

'Get up!' Linda said, taking a step back. 'Now!'

Linda gave her legs a little slap, tame in comparison to the treatment dished out to us but enough to startle our newest arrival. Reluctantly she got up, moved to the gap in the rail and slipped down to the floor.

'Now, if you're too hot, take off your nightie.'

Megan looked terrified. Even in the half-light I could see she was shaking. Was that how I looked when it dawned on me the girls had been right all along? What was Linda playing at?

'It's okay now,' Megan said, trembling, 'I'm not hot anymore.'

'Take off your nightie.' Linda's tone was controlled but menacing.

Megan did as she was told and slipped out of her nightdress. She hugged her semi-naked frame. With a deepening sense of unease I rolled to the edge of my pillow to get a better look and saw Linda walk to the table and pull out one of the chairs.

'Now come over here.'

Megan hesitated.

'Now!'

She shuffled over quickly.

'Stand on this.' Linda pointed to the chair.

What? This was new.

'Stand?' Megan said, looking confused.

'Stand on the chair!'

I almost couldn't watch. It was one thing to pick on us but we'd grown used to it. She didn't need to make an example of Megan. She'd soon learn – but maybe not fast enough for Linda's liking.

Megan climbed up onto the chair, holding on to the back for support, her knees bent, trying to be as small as possible, still trying to cover her modesty with her other hand.

'Stand up straight!'

If the tears hadn't been forming in Megan's eyes before they sure were now. I could hear her sniffing. I heard shuffling above me and imagined Sara was watching this unfold too. I could make out Arlene's unblinking eyes from over in her bunk.

'No holding on. Come on now, Megan, stand up straight on the chair.'

Very slowly Megan stood to her full height. She was now taller than Linda. She found her balance and stood with her hands clasped in front of her.

'Good,' Linda said, taking a step back as if to admire her handiwork. 'You can stay in that position while you think about how important it is to do as I say. Maybe next time when I tell you to be quiet, you'll listen. If I come back and you're not standing exactly like this you'll be in even more trouble. Understand?'

Megan nodded as a tear ran down her cheek. She managed to hold it together until Linda left the room and then the sobbing began. I sat up, horrified. Tormenting us older girls was one thing but this was taking things too far. She was shaking so much I thought she might fall from the chair. I got up and, holding a hand up for her to stay where she was, walked slowly and silently to the door. Focusing on me and wondering what I was up to distracted her enough for the sobbing and shaking to stop. I pointed to the other side of the door and put a finger to my lips. She nodded. I waited by the door for what seemed like eternity until finally I heard sounds that Linda had retreated downstairs. Then I went over to Megan. She jumped down.

'What are you doing? Get back on there. She'll be back soon and if you're not still there she'll go nuts.'

Megan wasn't listening. She picked up her nightie, put it on and climbed back into bed. Good for you, I thought. You'll suffer for it probably but at least you've got spunk.

It was only a few minutes later when Linda returned. I knew she wouldn't leave it too long. We were all expecting it. Just like we expected the fury.

'Did I say you could go back to bed?' she screamed, smacking Megan over the duvet.

Linda stopped short of dragging her out of bed and forcing her to perform her punishment again but the poor girl went without breakfast the following morning and her honeymoon period was well and truly over. That was it for her. She had become one of us. It was what she had always wanted – to be in our room – but this was probably not what she imagined.

We all knew that we needed to do something if we were to protect her from the type of beatings and punishment that we endured. For in May 2003, about a month before my fifteenth birthday, Megan got a taste of how brutal life in the Bad Room could be.

It was only 6 p.m. when Linda insisted we go to bed. Even by her standards this was early. There was no need for us to be completely silent, as Terry had only just returned home from work and we'd only just finished our dinner. I warned Megan about making things worse by talking so we resorted to passing notes instead. When Linda made her frequent visits to try to catch us out she had an inkling something was up but she couldn't put her finger on what. It was the following night that she found some of the notes we'd been passing. Megan had dropped one in among her sheets and Linda pounced after we'd been sent to bed. I didn't know which message she read but it was enough for her to drag Megan from her top bunk. Before any of us had time to react she hit her twice in the face. I couldn't watch. I turned away and heard five more slaps.

'Jade, what do you have to say about this?'

With Megan in tears, Linda bounded across brandishing the piece of paper. I tried to say it was nothing but she whacked me hard on the legs and back, the only parts of me she could reach before I wrapped the duvet around for protection.

When she stormed out we all calmed Megan down and I inspected my wounds. I had a mark on my back and legs. Megan's face was red raw and wet with tears.

'We have to do something about this,' I said. 'It can't go on.'

'What do we do?' Sara said.

'We need to tell our teachers. If we all do it and the schools tell the social workers, surely they have to do something?'

The following morning Linda seemed in a quieter mood as if she knew she'd overstepped the mark.

When I went into school I told my form teacher, Mrs O'Neill. I tried to show her the bruises from the night before but they had gone. Nevertheless, she took me seriously enough to call social services. My regular social worker, Claire, was on leave, but they sent someone else to speak to me at the school. Her name was Susan, a social worker I hadn't met before. I told her about the incidents involving Megan but also about Linda's general treatment of us – feeling like we were locked in our room, having to eat there, routinely being hit. I confessed I had been fearful of speaking out.

'I don't want to go back there tonight,' I said.

Susan spoke to Mrs O'Neill, who confirmed Sara had told another teacher the same story. When she came back she persuaded me to go home, basically because they were at a loss with what else to do. She said Brenda, who had carried out the investigation into Mum's report, and another social worker would meet us there. We arrived and I was sent upstairs while they spoke with Linda and Terry. I didn't have to be in the room to know what Linda would be saying. I could well imagine. She'd deny hitting any of us, she'd say I always made a fuss and this was attention seeking, just like the times I'd ran away.

Sure enough, their meeting ended with no drastic solutions being offered. The social workers left saying Linda would have a chat with me and I was to speak to them in the morning. All night I waited, expecting Linda to have it out with me, but she barely came into the room and when she did she refused to make eye contact. There was certainly not going to be any heart-to-heart.

In the morning all she said to me was, 'Well, Jade, what are you going to do? Do you still want to live here?'

What could I say? It was clear there was no appetite from social services to change anything.

I had to accept I was stuck there. I knew one thing, though: we would have to protect Megan from the worst of Linda's anger, to teach her how to avoid getting caught if she needed to go to the toilet and not to do things that needlessly provoked her violence. If we didn't Megan would discover what the rest of us had

– that when social services started to take less of an interest, you are on your own. We all desperately needed some respite from the unrelenting misery.

Chapter 21

It came out of the blue and it was bliss, like being on holiday. We could do what we wanted, go wherever we wanted, eat like normal people. It wasn't a dream. It was actually happening. And we loved it.

When Linda broke the news to us that she had to go into hospital for a hernia operation the implications didn't sink in at first.

'Terry will be looking after you,' she said before she left, 'so no mucking about. I want you to be on your best behaviour and don't give him any trouble.'

That's when we realised. Two days without Linda. Two days without being shouted at, without walking around on eggshells and without having to shower together. Even then it took a while for us to adjust. So conditioned were we to our routine that it was actually Megan who showed us we could just wander about without anyone questioning it.

Terry might have been at home to look after us but

he was hardly running a tight ship. He didn't just let us play outside, he expected it. 'So, you're going out, then?'

'Yes,' we said and were outside before another word was spoken.

When it was time for dinner he suggested he get chippy teas for us all. Not only that but we could go into the kitchen cupboards and help ourselves to food. We were in heaven. It felt like he spoiled us. In fact, he was treating us like normal children. He let us watch TV, play on Lisa's games consoles and hang out where we wanted. Although we could go to the toilet without having to be told, some things never changed. When it came to shower time we were so conditioned to life under Linda's rule that we still showered together, although not immediately after our dinner.

On the second day I went exploring through parts of the house I never got the chance to see. Sara and I went into the old dining room, where Linda stored all our Christmas presents. There they all were, gathering dust because she was too mean to let us have them for more than a week.

'Here, look at this,' Sara said. She was over at a cabinet stacked with ornamental plates. Behind one of the plates were letters. I went to investigate and, taking them from her, I caught my breath. They were from my mum. I couldn't quite believe it. There were several – letters that my mum had sent to social services and that they'd copied and forwarded on to Linda. I had never seen any of them before.

I turned them over in my hand, looking at her neat, arty handwriting. I almost wasn't sure if I should read them but the desire to see what she was saying was too much.

The one on the top said, 'I love you.' Mum said she had got a new house. She was living on the coast in Somerset. She said she was going to get us back and added, 'Please remember the good.'

In another she said 'I hope Linda's being nice.' I thought about how she'd reported Linda way back in the early days. Then I thought how Linda insulted my mum. As I read on, Mum said in the letter to tell Linda she was not a bad person. Reading her words knocked me sideways. Before then I'd never really bothered about my mum. She couldn't look after us and that was that. I kept playing her words over in my head: 'Remember the good.' The passing of the years had made that harder and harder. Were there any good times? I could only remember the bad.

I was more upset that my mum had written to me and Linda thought she wouldn't pass them on. When I finished reading them all I put them back the way they were. What else would we find? What else was Linda hiding from us?

We went to Lisa's room and started looking through her chest of drawers. Then my heart truly stopped.

Buried at the back of a drawer, underneath some clothes and junk, was my radio 'Walkman', the one Dad gave me on the last day I saw him. I was completely shocked. On one hand I was elated that I hadn't 'lost it' as Linda had always claimed. On the other I was sickened that she not only took it from me but also lied to make me feel bad. Were there no depths to which this woman would sink?

I was so tempted to take it and hide it in my room, but if she found it she would know I'd gone looking for it. As I did with the letters, I left it where it was. I retreated from the room with a hollow feeling in my stomach.

That night Terry again let us have free rein of the house. Over the two days I ate more than I had over the previous week, so much so I felt bloated and sick. I put it down to gorging where previously I had survived on meagre rations and didn't think much more about it.

When Linda came home from hospital she was fuming when she found out we were playing outside. 'You know you're not allowed to play outside.'

'Terry said it was okay,' I said.

'It seems you've been taking advantage of his good nature,' she scowled.

Still poorly after her operation, she announced that she would be bedridden for a week and it might take double that time for her to fully recuperate. As she was unable to walk, running up the stairs was out of the question, so our holiday from her usual tirade continued. So incapacitated was she that she asked Sara to go to the shops for her. When she did so, Sara kept a couple of pounds from the change in case it came in handy when we needed to eat once the starvation started again.

Rather than trying to impose her usual military regime, which she wouldn't be able to enforce, Linda wanted us to be occupied, so she let us watch TV. She was on strong medication so the less hassle the better. She sent Sara to the chip shop for dinner again so our treats continued, even though I still struggled to finish a big plateful.

We tried to be helpful by doing the cleaning and running Lisa's bath. We wanted to prove we could be responsible by going to bed at a sensible time and keeping the noise down without her shouting at us. Despite everything, we still wanted to please her.

For two nearly two weeks life in that house was bearable. We almost got used to coming home from school and not having to retreat immediately to our room. We didn't see Linda in the mornings so we just helped ourselves to breakfast and sorted our own lunches.

Every day I left for school I prayed for another day of bed rest for Linda. For a while those prayers were answered, until the day I came home and she was at the door to greet me.

'Oh, you're up,' I said. 'Feeling better?'

'A lot better, you'll be glad to know,' she said, that glint returning to her eye. 'Things can get back to normal around here.'

My heart sank. In a forlorn hope that her recovery might have led to a change in attitude from her I asked if there was anything we could do to help, like get dinner.

'No, thank you. I'm fine,' she said, 'just make yourself scarce and I'll call you for dinner as usual.'

She might not have been able to get up the stairs as fast as she could before but she wanted to show us she was still in charge. After our tea she was on shower patrol, handing out dollops of shampoo as before. Her operation might have diminished her ability to dish out physical attacks but she more than made up for that with verbal assaults instead.

As we stripped off for showers, her eyes scanned our bodies, looking for anything to pick fault with. I was self-conscious enough about my figure. At 14 I was skinny from malnutrition but had large 34E breasts, which I always feared looked weird on my size-ten frame. The last thing I wanted was anyone pointing this out, which of course Linda did.

'I swear you're turning into quite the fat slag with that chest of yours,' she sneered. She also singled me out for my olive skin and green eyes, calling me 'Paki eyes'.

'You could be mistaken for a Turkish Muslim,' she quipped while eyeing me up and down. 'I bet all your little girlfriends love you, you dyke. Don't they? I bet you're a right little lesbian.'

Hearing comments like that made me want to die. I hated undressing for PE, fearing that other girls must think the same as she did when they saw my body. I was ashamed of my appearance and tried to hide my chest when I could. The recent bloated feeling didn't help. Although there was nothing to me, aside from my chest, I felt fat and unfit.

Despite the love of dance I'd had when I was younger, for over four years since moving into Linda's house I hadn't done one class. She'd banned us from any extra-curricular activities. When I'd asked about doing dancing she'd said: 'You'd never be any good as a dancer. Your legs are too fat and you're too chubby to do that.' As a result, any passion for physical exercise had been sapped from me. I was approaching my fifteenth birthday and I felt horrible and ugly.

It wasn't just me she targeted with her abuse. They say children are cruel but I'd never met anyone so adept at picking on a person's insecurities.

'You're quite the Paki as well,' she said to Arlene during our shower sessions. 'How come you both look like that? Were your mums both done by a Paki? I bet that's it. Your mums got done by a Paki and that's why you two are now Pakis.'

Such verbal taunts cut us to the bone but they also sickened us to the point where we rebelled.

While Linda had been in hospital, we'd built up a bit of a rapport with Lisa again, playing in her room and watching movies with her. Now Linda was out we tried to use that to our advantage.

'Go downstairs and ask your mum to put a film on – and say you'd like us to watch it with you,' we said to her, 'but don't tell her we asked you.'

Lisa would do so and through this low-level deception we got to watch some films, like the *Harry Potter* movies she was obsessed with. It was a small victory in an otherwise unrelenting battle of wits.

As Linda got stronger and resumed her attempts to catch us out at night-time, the more we joined forces to frustrate her. We schooled Megan in the ways of the Bad Room so she became better at avoiding getting caught. Sara and Arlene showed her how to get to the toilet avoiding the squeakiest of floorboards. Both sisters had grown into quite gangly teenagers and I found it funny watching them straddle the hallway, legs wide apart, their feet practically touching the skirting boards on each side of the carpet. We told her about using the bidet, how never to pull the flush and to drink direct from the tap without spilling water down the plughole. We showed her the paper in the door and taught her how to remove it and replace without being detected.

If Linda did hear any of us talking and stormed into the room she was met with a wall of silence. Gone were the days when someone would squeal on the culprit in a bid to win favour. We were in this together. We had each other's backs, looking out for each other. If one was down we picked her up and dusted her off to get her going again. If one was punished, we all got punished. For the first time in my life I was learning what girl friendship was all about. It made life a little more bearable for all of us.

One of the most remarkable transformations was Sara. I remembered her in my early days in the house, when she was so quiet and compliant. Softer than Arlene and me, she had always just wanted an easy life and couldn't help being a telltale. Now nearly 16, she wasn't afraid to look Linda in the eye and challenge her: 'Who do you think was talking? I heard no one.'

Linda, after years of relying on her to tell the truth, was regularly left flummoxed, forced to hit out randomly at whoever she thought was most culpable.

On the days that Linda refused to give us lunch, Sara used the money she'd stolen from the shopping trips to buy chocolate bars. These we snuck home and hid behind the bed, where the legs of the bunks went into an alcove. We'd wedge one behind the leg of the bunk beds and the wall and share it between us. On other days, if Sara had enough money, she'd buy a bar in the shop behind the school and the two of us ate it on the way home.

Linda was so suspicious she started checking us when we came in the door to see if we'd been buying food at school. Ordering us to leave our backpacks downstairs she told us to get up to the room while she rooted through our things for evidence of any other food. So convinced was she that we might be smuggling food into the house that she strip-searched us as we came in to check we weren't hiding anything.

She didn't find food but on one occasion she found something else. I'd chosen art as one of my GCSE subjects but I needed pencils to complete my course-work. Linda wouldn't give me the money for them so out of desperation I stole some from the classroom. Fearing a search of my bag, I tucked them in the top of my skirt under my jumper. My heart sank when she ordered us to strip that day. As soon as I lifted my jumper up they fell out.

A look of satisfaction came over her face. I just knew she'd tell the school, helping to reinforce her picture of me as a good-for-nothing tearaway. She also punished me by sending me to bed with no dinner. I was grateful for the small bits of chocolate that night.

I actually started to care less, though, about whatever treatment Linda dished out.

Sit me naked in the cold? I've already done it for 12 hours or more – and I survived. You want me to starve? I've been there already. I've learned to distract myself from the hunger pains and cramps. I can survive that. You want to beat me and knock me down? I know I can get back up. I can survive whatever you do to me. That's what I thought. I am a survivor.

One night, after I'd turned 15 and we'd gone back to school following the summer holidays, I felt like I'd been punished so often it was almost a miracle if I got my three meals a day. I'd been so used to going without I'd forgotten what I'd lost in the first place. I didn't care if she heard me open the door. I walked down the middle of the hall, setting off the squeaking floorboards. I did the toilet and pulled the flush, listening to it gurgle down the pipes, knowing it would lift her from the sofa and have her labouring up the stairs. I could still be back in the room before her, diving under the covers while she struck out at me.

'You horrible fat Paki,' she yelled at me.

'I'm going to tell my head of year that you've hit me,' I shouted from under the covers. 'I'll tell them all what you're like. Then you'll be sorry.'

'No one will believe you,' I heard her shout. 'You're a liar and a thief – and the school knows that.'

'I hate you!' I said, still buried under the duvet. 'I wish I was anywhere else but here.'

'No one would have you, Jade. You think another foster carer is going to want a manipulating, scheming and thieving little liar like you? I'm the only one who was ever willing to take you in.'

I pulled the covers from over my head so I could look her in the eye. Did she really believe that? 'That's not true,' I yelled.

Her contorted face was an ugly mix of rage and glee at the things she was saying. 'You leave here and there's only one place you're going, Jade – a children's home! Then you'll see how bad things really are. They are horrible places, full of nasty children, who no one wants. You don't know how good you've got it here. Social services know what I have to put up with here. You think it's so bad? Wait until you spend a week in a children's home with the rest of the horrible children that no one wants.'

'That's not true!' I shouted. Surely she was lying?

'Just try telling your teachers what you think goes on here – and see what happens. You're just a fat little Paki who no one wants to give a home to.'

Previously I might have cried on hearing such vitriol but I just buried my head under the duvet once more.

'Go away!' I shouted.

Cocooned under the covers I could hear her cackling laughter. She actually enjoyed saying stuff like that. Burning with rage, I would have loved to have hit out or done something back to her, but I just lay there, knowing that eventually she would leave the room.

It took me a long time to calm down after that shouting match. Over and over I replayed it in my head, scarcely able to believe what she had come out with.

Maybe she was right about one thing. I couldn't tell anyone what she said. Who would believe me?

Was it true what she said about no other foster carer wanting to take me? Was Linda the only option I had? Could she send me to a children's home?

I had no idea, but as the anger burned inside me I just thought I couldn't take it anymore. I'd had enough. Do your worst, I thought. Come on, really try to hurt me. See if I care.

I needed to be careful what I wished for, though, because one day she would do just that.

Chapter 22

As soon as I pulled the trousers over my knees I knew they weren't going to fit. I was gutted. Ever since I'd started the new school year I'd been desperate to get out of my school skirt. They relaxed the rules for older pupils and from Year 10 upwards girls were allowed to wear trousers.

Maybe Linda had felt the pressure from social services' visits but come October 2003 she finally bought me some new clothes to wear. I was excited at the prospect of wearing pants, as we all called them. It was a chance to be cool, a chance to fit in. I checked the size. They were a 12. That's why. She'd got the wrong size. They were too wide at the waist and slid down my hips. Was that on purpose? She always said I was bigger than I thought. Was this her way of telling me?

Lisa came through to watch me try them on. Although overweight, she was obsessed with everyone else's size and regularly taunted Arlene and Sara that they were fatter than she was. Clearly that wasn't the case. Both sisters were skinny and didn't eat enough to put on weight. Somehow Lisa got it into her head that they were, though.

When she saw the pants fall off me she started laughing. 'Why don't they fit her? Is that 'cos she's fat?'

'It's not because I'm fat,' I said, already annoyed. 'They're too big not too small.'

'Ha ha, look, Mum, Jade's fatter than me.'

Lisa was a sweet soul, normally, but she could also be annoying.

'Be quiet, will you,' I snapped. 'I'm not fat.'

Linda shrugged. 'That's the size. If they don't fit, just hang them up.'

Lisa picked them up. 'Jade's too fat,' she kept saying.

I grabbed them off her to put on a hanger, opened the wardrobe door and reached inside.

'Oi, don't snatch from her,' Linda shouted.

Suddenly my arm exploded in pain. She had slammed the wardrobe door on it.

'Ow!' I yelled.

I couldn't pull out my arm because Linda still held the door shut, trapping it. She opened the door and I tried to pull it out but she closed it on my arm again. The pain was excruciating. Again I tried to remove it. Again she trapped it in the door. I yelled again and it opened enough for me to free it. I pulled it to me at last, shaking in pain and fear. For a moment everything paused. We all stood stunned, taking in what had happened. I think even Linda was shocked by the suddenness and ferocity of her own violence. Lisa looked gobsmacked. I lifted my sleeve. My arm was red raw. I couldn't help the tears coming. I couldn't remember experiencing pain like it.

Linda still stood looking like she wasn't sure how to react. I dived over to my bed for refuge. 'I can't believe you did that. You could have broken it!' I cried, nursing it as best I could.

Lisa's hand was to her mouth. Linda still looked as though she was processing all the implications of this. A slightly scared look came over her face. Not for long. Then it curled into a snarl.

My school shoes were at the end of the bed. She picked one up and launched it through the bunk bed at me. I ducked and it bounced harmlessly away.

'It's your fault!' she screamed. 'You made me do it. You shouldn't have snatched them from Lisa like that. It's always your fault.'

Ushering Lisa out of the room, she followed her and slammed the door closed behind her. My arm throbbed. I curled up into a ball and cried myself to sleep.

When I woke, it took me a moment to remember what happened. Had I dreamt it? Then the burning, throbbing pain in my arm brought it all back. I inspected the injury. My upper arm was purple and black, my eyes were swollen and red.

I felt emotionally broken. I hated my looks, my body, every little aspect of me. Even the beauty spots on my face were picked on by Linda. I hardly said a word to anyone before I left the house. There was a heavy atmosphere, as though everyone could sense a line had been crossed. I only saw Linda once. She tried to look defiant but in her eyes I could detect some unease.

As I walked to school through the park I couldn't see a way out. This was never going to stop. There was no point reporting her or running away, as I always got sent back. I couldn't win against this woman. I felt defeated. I felt numb. I didn't want to be here anymore.

When I got to school I waited behind to let everyone into class. I didn't want anyone to see my puffy eyes. I wanted to get into the toilet and compose myself before attempting to go to class. It was 9.30 a.m. when I ventured inside school.

By pure chance I saw Leanne hurrying in. She was running late.

'What happened?' she said as soon as she saw me.

I led her to the toilet and showed her my arm.

'Oh my God,' she said when she saw the state of it.

I wanted to be strong but I couldn't help crying. I just felt so destitute. It didn't seem to matter the circumstances, Linda was always going to be horrible. I felt utterly broken, now physically as well as emotionally.

At least I had Leanne, who comforted and stayed with me while I sorted myself out and washed my face so my eyes could return to some sort of normality.

'You need to tell someone,' she said.

'I can't. No one believes me. It never makes a difference.' I thought about what Linda had said before about no one wanting me and if I left her the only place I'd be going to was a children's home.

We didn't share the same classes so Leanne and I went our separate ways, promising to meet up once the school day was over. I got my head down and just tried to concentrate on my lessons.

It was nearing the end of the day, at about 3 p.m., when Mr Jones, a head of year teacher, appeared in my English class, asking if he could have a word with me. Oh no, I thought, I must be in trouble. Why was Mr Jones involved? He wasn't one of my heads of year so it was strange he was getting me out of class. My mind raced with the possibilities. Had Linda rung the school? If so, what had she said? Was I going to a home?

When we got to his office, he showed me to a seat, sat down and said, 'Are you okay?'

'Yes,' I said, still trying to work out what was going on.

'How's your home life?'

'Fine.' I could feel my usual guard come up. It was like those very first days of primary school, when teachers quizzed me about my mum. 'Why?'

'Can you roll your sleeve up please?'

'No.' What was going on?

'Please, can you just roll your sleeve up,' he said. His tone was soft. It didn't seem like I was in trouble but I couldn't be sure. 'It's all right, everything will be all right.'

Slowly I rolled up my sleeve. My arm was still bruised, now purple and yellow. Seeing it brought back the image and pain of when the door smashed into it.

He took a moment to look at it, his brow furrowed. 'Right, you're not going home today. This is going to be sorted out.'

What? Did I just hear right? I wasn't going home? If I wasn't, where was I going?

'Your friend brought this to the school's attention,' Mr Jones said.

Leanne. Of course. She didn't even tell me she was going to do anything. Mr Jones slipped out of the room to speak to another teacher. I just sat there, trying to process what was happening. The door was ajar behind me but I was aware of someone standing there. I turned. It was Sara. Just then Mr Jones returned. He gestured to her to come in.

'What are you doing?' she said. 'I was waiting for you outside. Leanne told me you were in here.'

'I don't know,' I said. 'I just got called out of class.'

'Sara, you'll need to go home as usual,' Mr Jones told her. 'We're notifying Mrs Black but Jade won't be coming home.'

Sara looked stunned. 'Linda's going to go ballistic,' she said.

She was right. Mr Jones better be right about me not having to go home to face her. If this led to nothing, as usual, I was in big trouble.

Mr Jones was on the phone to Linda. I could just imagine what story she was spinning – how it was my entire fault. 'Mrs Black, you're a liar,' I heard him say. Oh my God!

'We've got records,' he went on. 'Jade won't be stepping foot in that fucking house again.' I couldn't believe it. Did he really say that? The anger in his voice and the fact that he swore took me aback.

When he came off the phone, he filled me in on what she had said. According to her I'd got into a fight with one of the other girls and that's what caused the bruising. I felt scared. If that's what she was saying, what did it mean?

Next he rang social services. It sounded like they were trying to get him to return me to Linda, saying they would sort it out – just like they did after Megan and I were hit. I might have known. My heart started to sink. I had been here before.

But he was adamant. 'No, you can come and get her now, she's not returning to that house.'

Mr Jones explained to me after that the school had been keeping a file on me. Although I hadn't given them the full story of what life was like at Linda's they kept a record of all the incidents – when she pulled my hair out, the times she'd hit me, when I'd resorted to stealing to buy something to eat. It transpired they also kept tabs on Sara's situation. When Leanne told them about the latest incident and they saw my bruises they felt they had to act. He explained they would send Sara home as usual but they would speak to social services about us all. Sara seemed okay with this. I hoped that, because of what was happening with me, Linda would be extra nice to her and Arlene. Maybe things would be bearable for them and it wouldn't be long before action was taken with them too.

I had to wait around while social services worked out a plan. I was relieved to see it was Claire, my regular social worker, who arrived to deal with me. She quickly dispelled any concern I had that she would return me to Linda. In fact, she was happy I wasn't going back there.

'We're going to find you someone to stay with on a short-term emergency basis until we work out a longer-term plan,' she said. 'I'm sorry this has gone on so long, Jade. It might not seem like it but we were trying to find a solution. At least this incident has forced action to happen.'

After another long wait, Claire confirmed that a woman called Yvonne, who had been my brother's foster carer for a while, was able to take me and was coming to pick me up. I'd always thought she was lovely so I couldn't be happier. It was all very surreal. Was this really happening? I felt elated, buzzing. Were people finally listening to me? Were they actually accepting that what I was saying was the truth? It was an amazing feeling. After five years was I finally getting away from Linda?

'Come on, before we go home, let's go and get you some things,' Yvonne said, once we set off. The only belongings I had were the clothes on my back and my school bag.

Yvonne took me to a late-night Asda. She picked up food for our dinner. It was amazing to be given choice and the thought of a cooked meal made my mouth water.

'Let's find you some pyjamas to wear,' Yvonne said as she led me to the clothes section. Pyjamas! Was she serious? For five years I'd worn the same nightie that was now so small I couldn't even get it over my knees. To be faced with a rack of nightclothes and asked to choose something was mind blowing.

'Go on,' she said, seeing my hesitation. 'You can choose something. Claire told me to get things for you. It's all okay.'

It was so exciting. I picked a new pyjama set and felt like a kid in a sweet shop. She let me choose some other clothes so I had something to change into the next day. Having a say in what I wanted to wear was such an alien concept for me. I almost didn't know where to begin.

'What shall I get?'

By the look on Yvonne's face I think she was only now getting a sense of how restrictive my life had been. She kindly helped me to pick something and then took me to the audio section.

'As I treat why don't you choose yourself a CD?'

Was she serious? I almost wanted to cry. It was as if she knew how important music was to me. Emotions I'd buried for so long threatened to bubble to the surface. In a flash I was taken back to the days spent singing and dancing to my mum's tunes and to the comfort I got from listening to the radio on my dad's Walkman. During those years of enforced silence at Linda's, the only music I'd been able to listen to was if Lisa had the TV on or if my friends talked about a new artist they were into. I felt a whole generation of pop music had passed me by.

I chose Dido's new album *Life for Rent*. She had been one of those acts that I'd been vaguely aware of but had missed out on when she went massive. After a long break she was back on the scene with a new album that had only just been released. It seemed fitting.

Our shopping trip over, Yvonne took me to her house. Once inside, I stood there, not knowing what to do, waiting to be ordered somewhere.

'Just relax,' she said. 'I'll get you something to eat and you can have a shower. What a stressful day, you must be exhausted.'

Yvonne had a grown-up son and daughter, both in their early twenties. They couldn't have been more welcoming. Her daughter Pamela put on the CD for me and showed me their music collection. Her brother was a musician and in a band so they had loads of CDs. There were acts that my mum loved, like Madonna.

'Listen to anything you want,' Pamela said.

Yvonne had a downstairs shower and in her bedroom was an ensuite bathroom with a shower over the bath.

She handed me a towel and my new pyjamas and showed me into her ensuite. 'There you go,' she said, 'help yourself to anything you need. Lock the door, give yourself some privacy and take as long as you want.'

'Thank you,' I said, clutching my stuff.

She closed the door and left me inside. I slid the lock over, scarcely believing what I was doing. Was I really in a bathroom by myself? With a shower I could use without someone standing there, watching, making comments about my body? And the shampoo bottles? Could I really be trusted to put some on my hair myself?

For a few moments I just stood there, looking around, half expecting her to come back in and say, 'Actually it's all been a mistake, you're going back to Linda's.'

Slowly, I put down my things and ran the shower. The bathroom smelled so nice and the warm mist so inviting. When I finally stepped in I just stood for a few minutes letting the warm water wash over me. I closed my eyes and kept telling myself, 'this is real, this is actually happening.' I must have stood under that shower for half an hour, just enjoying being on my own, with no one shouting or listening by the door.

This must be what heaven feels like, I thought.

Dressed in my new cosy PJs, tucked into a warm bed in a lovingly decorated room, I felt so happy. Was my ordeal really over? As I lay awake a faint sense of unease came over me. What was I scared of? I thought about the girls back in the Bad Room. Hopefully they would have had a nice evening too. A proper meal, maybe even getting to watch some television? Surely Linda would be on her best behaviour? But what if she wasn't? What if things were as bad as always? What if, in the time I had been with Yvonne, Linda had been peddling her lies and convincing social services to send me back? Don't be silly, I told myself, everyone said you don't have to go back there. Why then did I feel that Linda still had the ability to hurt me?

Chapter 23

Just when I thought I was safe the door flew open. I couldn't make out her face but there she was, standing in the door, silhouetted against the light. I ducked under the covers but she was too quick for me, wrenching the duvet from my grasp. My tiny threadbare nightie offered zero protection as she lashed out again and again on my legs, back and head.

'No, no, please no,' I cried, my ears ringing to the sound of her cackling laughter.

And then it was over. I woke up with a start and was shocked to see the duvet still over me, a plump pillow behind my head. There was no nightie, I was in the pyjamas Yvonne had bought me.

It was just a dream. A horrible nightmare.

The door opened. I gasped and shrank back. It was Yvonne.

'It's okay, it's okay, you've had another nightmare. You were screaming out.' She cuddled me in her arms and sat with me until I dozed off.

In my early days at Yvonne's house that happened a lot. I might have escaped Linda's physical clutches but the emotional scars would take much longer to heal, if they ever did.

Those dreams apart, though, life at Yvonne's could not have been a greater contrast to the life I'd known. She was chilled, she didn't shout and she didn't make unreasonable demands.

'You know when you're tired and need to go to bed,' she said, when it got near bedtime. She let me go to sleep listening to music. My bedroom was now my sanctuary. I liked to go upstairs, light the candles and listen to music for hours. But I also loved spending time getting to know her family. Her daughter Pamela cuddled me on the sofa while we watched TV together. She taught me how to put on make-up and style my hair, things other teenagers learn as a rite of passage and take for granted. Meanwhile, Yvonne's son John showed me some basic chords on the guitar.

When I first moved to Yvonne's, I didn't go to school for the rest of that week. Claire told me they'd asked Linda to pass my clothes and belongings to the school but she had only dropped in a few bits and pieces. I wasn't too bothered about my clothes as I hardly had any, but I had coursework at her house for my GCSE, including an art portfolio I'd spent a lot of time building and she claimed wasn't at her house.

I was gutted. It meant I would have to do it all again. Even though she couldn't reach me she still found ways to hurt me.

Yvonne took me shopping again and bought me new school clothes and PE kit, items that actually fitted me. By the time I went back to school I felt a different girl. Like nearly everyone my age, I was allowed to wear a little make-up and actually had clothing that wasn't the cheapest, most easily identifiable non-brand gear that kids immediately pounce on for not being fashionable.

Yvonne gave me £20 and trusted me to use it to buy school lunches. She also said I could meet my friends after school. The feeling of freedom was amazing. Bumping into Sara for the first time since leaving the house was a strange experience. I'd been thinking of them all constantly, hoping that life had improved for them or that they too had been moved to someone who would actually care for them. Given the horrible circumstances in which we'd met and bonded, I missed being with them, yet I was also so glad to be free. As she approached me, however, the look on her face said everything.

'Look at you,' she said. 'You're so different. What's going on?'

I filled her in on how life had been at Yvonne's house. She looked enviously at my hair and nails and I felt a little guilty telling her about the freedom I'd already experienced and had been promised.

'How are things with Linda?'

'Not bad,' she shrugged. 'Bit better. We get to watch TV. And we get our meals.'

There was a bit of a silence and awkwardness between us.

'Are you coming back? She asked me to find out. She wants to see you,' Sara said. 'She told me to tell you to go up to the house and speak to her. She wants to sort it out.'

I felt bad for her and the others still stuck there. Clearly social services saw no problem keeping them there. If the school hadn't stepped in on my behalf I'd be there still. Perhaps Sara hadn't made any specific complaints about her own treatment and that had made it difficult for the school to intervene. The thought of going and speaking to Linda turned my stomach. Did I really want to go back there and see her again? It had all ended suddenly, almost surreally. Should I do the right thing and hear what she had to say?

I told Sara I'd try to go up the next day. My only chance would be to sneak out of school at lunchtime, as after school Yvonne collected me in her car. I didn't want to tell anyone what I was doing. I hadn't even convinced myself it was a good idea. I was only really doing it for Sara.

The following lunchtime I snuck out of school and walked the familiar route to Linda's. Normally I trudged the pavements like a condemned prisoner.

Now it felt strange to have some degree of power and control. It would only be a brief meeting and when it was over I could leave. But when I turned into the road that led to the house my tummy started churning. This was the point at which Sara and I usually parted in case she was watching. I had a sense of dread. Something told me this was not a good idea.

Arriving at the door, Linda welcomed me like a long-lost relative. 'So good to see you. What's going on? What are you doing with Yvonne?'

It was so weird to see her like this, even being there on these terms – me, as a visitor, rather than her prisoner. My emotions were in turmoil. I felt guilty, scared, but also empowered. She had made me believe I was a bad girl, that I couldn't be trusted and couldn't live a normal life. I wanted to prove her wrong. I wanted to show her I was worthy of a normal teenage life.

I composed myself and began to fill her on what had happened at Yvonne's and told her that I could go out and play in the streets.

'Ah, but the reason you can't do that here,' she butted in, 'is because you can't be trusted.'

'Trusted for what?' I said. 'You never trusted me and I've never done anything wrong.'

Linda brushed over that and changed the subject by offering to make lunch. I couldn't believe it when I saw that it was a ham sandwich – the very thing I'd had most in the last five years.

For the remainder of my time in the house she repeated her usual promises, that if I came back all would be different, I'd get to wear make-up, see my friends, watch more TV, go to bed later. I listened to her without saying much.

'Come back,' she said, when it was time for me to leave. 'Have a think about it and I'll sort it out. I'll fix it with social services and everything will be all right.'

For the briefest of seconds she almost seduced me with her talk of how she'd change and she'd do things the way Yvonne did. Then I thought of the sandwich and the memories came back of all the times I'd been stuck in the Bad Room and I thought, no. This is not the life for me. That sandwich showed nothing was going to change.

I saw Sara the next day and told her, 'No. You can tell her I'm not coming back.'

Perhaps understandably, she got angry at that. 'It's going to be bad now for the rest of us if you don't. You know it will.'

I was inclined to agree with her. I knew what she was like, after all. Surely, though, she could see I had to look after myself. This was a chance for me. I'd got out. There was no way I wanted to be sucked back in.

She stormed off and it saddened me to think our friendship might not survive me leaving. We had been through so much together, kindred souls in a nightmarish situation. I hoped she'd come round once things settled down but the only times she spoke to me in the weeks that followed were to give me little updates on life in the house.

'You're making Linda ill,' she said one day. 'Her hernia is bad.'

'I'm sorry to hear that,' I said, and I meant it, although I hoped that meant things were a bit calmer for them all. 'You look different,' I added. Sara appeared to be wearing make-up.

'Linda lets me wear it now,' she said. 'She also gives me dinner money. And she lets me have a smoke with her.'

It was obvious Linda was doing everything to keep Sara onside. I'd suspected Sara had smoked before but I was shocked to hear that.

'She buys me cigarettes,' she added, looking a bit pleased.

I wanted her to be happy. I wasn't sure that was the best way to go about it, but if seeing me have a bit of freedom had changed Linda's mindset then that had to be a good thing, surely? It was funny though. It almost felt as though she was competing with Yvonne. I didn't care. I liked living with Yvonne. During meetings I had with my social worker, Claire, she said an alternative arrangement for my care had not been found so, as long as I was content to stay with her, I could. I was delighted.

I worried for Sara. In the short interactions we had since I'd left the house, it was like she had become warped by Linda. She tried to pass on messages from her begging me to see her, that she wasn't well and wanted to talk about what had happened. This messed with my mind. I could sense it was affecting my mental health. I didn't want to know how ill Linda was. I wanted to forget I had ever met her, but it was proving impossible.

Claire kept updating me with events in my old house. Only a few weeks after I left, social services removed Arlene from Linda's care. I hadn't seen her since the morning of the day I left. In the period since then she had kicked off with her social worker that she didn't want to stay there any longer. They removed her and only a few short weeks after that they found a new home for Sara, too. I was glad they were finally out of there. That left only poor Megan in the house on her own, with just Lisa for company. Knowing how sociable she was I felt for her and hoped she was coping. I thought it strange that they could move three children amid allegations of ill-treatment yet leave a younger child in her care. This situation became even more remarkable when Claire told me social services had reviewed the claims made by Arlene, Sara and me, and felt there were grounds to involve the police and potentially have Linda charged for assaulting us.

'What do you think about that?' Claire asked me. 'Would you want to press charges against her?'

'What would happen to her?' I asked.

'She could possibly go to prison,' Claire said. 'These are serious allegations. The courts take a dim view on carers who assault children.'

I thought of this old woman, with her health problems, languishing in prison. What good would it serve? As long as no children were being made to feel like I had surely that was enough? I knew Megan was still there but, if Sara was to be believed, life there was not half as bad as before, with Linda not well enough to impose her cruelty.

'No,' I said to her. 'I've left now. I'm never going back. It's done with.'

In my immediate future I had a lot of hard work to do for my GCSEs. Linda never did return my coursework, either for art or English. In one of our infrequent conversations, Sara told me she had seen my art portfolio in the dining room, yet Linda swore to social services she had handed it in.

Claire tried to get other items belonging to me from the house. Of most importance was a journal on my brother and sister, including photos of them during the time we'd been apart. That was also mysteriously lost. Social services wouldn't go into the house to demand my things back. Claire just said, 'We've called her for it.'

In the absence of my coursework I had eight weeks to get four years' worth of work done. I was up all night at Yvonne's, making endless cups of coffee to stay awake, to make up the lost work. I ended up getting lower grades in art and English than I would have got but at least I passed.

Once my exams were out of the way I was free to take advantage of the new privileges Yvonne gave me. If I'm honest it was too much too soon. I got my first job in McDonald's when I turned 16, got my first mobile phone and had my first night out – which perhaps inevitably led to me getting drunk for the first time. After years of living such a restricted life I couldn't handle having so much freedom. I stayed out late and slept in.

I left school for a sixth-form college nearby to do performing arts, which included singing, acting and, in my second year, a dance course. It was a chance to reconnect with a passion that had been quashed for five years.

I felt like I had a lot of catching up to do and in that first year away from Linda I struggled to cope. I struggled with my sexuality, got into a relationship that wasn't healthy, and had no idea what was acceptable and what wasn't.

I'd had nothing for years and then a sensory overload and I didn't know how to deal with it. I also didn't know how to deal with the emotional scars from five years of mental and physical abuse.

All those years of being starved took their toll, too. From day one Yvonne treated me kindly and there was always food available to me to eat. By giving me money to spend and then when I had my own income, I was able to treat myself. Yet, although I could put those days of going hungry behind me, the memories weren't as easy to shake. I couldn't see it at first but my legacy of the abuse was cripplingly low self-esteem, a hatred of food and a hatred of my body – a dangerous combination under any circumstances.

Put simply, I had an unhealthy relationship with food. I was eating but trying desperately to control what I ate. Although I could have what I wanted I still restricted myself. I limited my intake to one meal a day. Just one. It didn't matter what Yvonne or my friends said, I wouldn't eat any more than that. I was in control. I'd skip a day and go to college and only drink water, and the next day I'd have a steak and salad and whatever Yvonne made for me. She spotted a pattern and informed my social worker. She tried to speak to me but my guard came up, I got defensive and only told her what I thought she wanted to hear.

I was losing weight but going out at the weekend drinking alcopops filled with sugar. I went through stages of wanting to be in control and other times not really caring, suffering the consequences. Some weekends I stayed out for two or three nights, mostly crashing with friends, but not telling Yvonne where I was, which only caused her and her family worry. She tried to reach out to me, as did my social worker, but I thought I could handle it.

I also thought I could handle it when completely unexpectedly my mum got in touch with social services. She wanted to see me. The social workers were wary. I hadn't seen her in five years and they were worried what impact resuming contact after all that time would do to me.

I was curious, though – curious to see what she looked like, hear what she had to say. I had heard she was taking steps to remain clean of drugs, but I'd heard that before. A meeting was arranged near to where we used to live. Mum was back living in a city many miles away so it was considered a neutral venue. I had my social worker with me and she counselled me before the meeting. There were certain things I couldn't discuss, like the whereabouts of my siblings. I'd resumed contact with them since leaving Linda's care and it had been wonderful to catch up with them, but due to conditions attached to our various care orders I had to keep the details to myself.

We met and Mum gave me a big hug. She had said she was clean of drugs but I remembered the signs from when I was a young girl. She might be off heroin but she was clearly still on methadone.

When we spoke, Mum sounded like she had in the letters I'd found in Linda's dining room. She wanted to control my thoughts on what happened in the past and how I now viewed her. 'Remember the good times,' she kept saying.

I just nodded, as another disturbing memory flashed in my mind.

Mum revealed she had been diagnosed with schizophrenia. I felt sorry for her because whatever had gone wrong in her life, that was something she had to live with.

I thought about asking her questions that had been playing on my mind for five years, like why she did what she did, why she behaved in a certain way, why she allowed her children to be taken off her? But as I looked at her I realised that none of that was going to sink in. She was still working through her troubles, so why add to them? I tried to be warm, and we left on good terms, but I came away with yet more conflicting emotions.

In the weeks following our visit I spiralled into depression – but I didn't heed the warning signs. I was behaving recklessly, believing I was enjoying life but really I was on a self-destructive path.

Mostly I was angry, preferring to dwell on what I'd lost rather than what I had. I didn't see myself as a newly confident teenager with my life ahead of me; able to focus on the things I loved doing. Instead I saw the girl Linda said I was. Convinced I was fat, I hated my large breasts. No amount of exercise or dancing seemed to change my body shape. I felt I was stuck with a body I despised.

My emotions got the better of me. I had no way of dealing with the turmoil inside me. Although I no longer had to hear Linda's cruel name-calling, in my head I still had those insecurities. I felt like I didn't belong in this world, that I'd been denied basic things that most people took for granted – like the unconditional love from their family. When I looked back on the events that had brought me to this situation I heard Linda's voice when she said, 'It is all your fault.' What if she was right? I thought of Mum and her toxic relationship with Paul, all the constant fighting, his dislike of me because I wasn't his, her mood swings when he wasn't around. Maybe I was the cause of everyone's unhappiness? I thought of my dad and how the contact had dried up. He hadn't wanted me in his life, it seemed.

With all these thoughts swirling around in my head, the only conclusion I could draw was that I wanted to sleep. I wanted the memories to switch off and the destructive negative feelings to disappear. I wanted to take back control. The only way to achieve this, I decided, was to take matters into my own hands.

Chapter 24

The razor blade hovered above my wrist. One cut might be all it would take. I wasn't consciously thinking about ending it all, I just wanted to stop the negative thoughts replaying endlessly in my head. This way I was in control. It was my decision.

Something stopped me. I couldn't physically push the blade into my wrist. Maybe I didn't want to die, maybe I didn't want the scars if I wasn't successful. Maybe I thought the sight of myself sitting there, razor blade in hand, might shock me out of the malaise in which I found myself. I don't know.

It did have some effect, though. I knew that this wasn't the answer. The potential violence of such an act scared me. I pulled back from that most decisive course of action. But the thoughts still remained. The desire to switch off the memories that haunted me and the feelings of worthlessness were still very much there.

And so I turned to paracetamol. Lots of them. I just wanted to sleep and not to feel and not to think about what happened. I had been away from Linda for a year but I hadn't dealt with anything that happened in those five years I had spent with her. I should have had counselling for my low self-esteem, my body image, the names she used to call us. I had an erratic eating pattern. There were lots of things I should've got help for but I didn't. If there was help available maybe social services should have been more forceful in telling me about it. Maybe I should have been more open to the idea. It didn't matter. This was where I found myself. I was quite happy to take a load of pills knowing I wasn't going to wake up. I was comfortable with that.

I remember drifting off. The next thing I knew I was in hospital, where a doctor told me I was lucky. Yvonne had found me in time. She came into my room, saw me asleep and saw the empty boxes. She roused me enough to take me to hospital where I now was. 'If you take that many paracetamol you're going to die a painful death,' the doctor said.

Shocked that I taken things this far and feeling so guilty that I had caused Yvonne so much worry, it was the wake-up call I needed. I didn't want to die, I just wanted to sleep. I just didn't want to think about what had happened. I still wanted some degree of control over the demons that tormented me, but I realised that taking a whole packet of paracetamol was not the way to do it.

When I thought about the things I could change, the factor that caused me the most grief was that I couldn't escape the feelings around my body. The hatred I felt for my figure – in particular the breasts I felt were over-sized for my shape – represented everything I felt about food and the horrible memories of Linda's cruel taunts. The more I thought about it the more I realised that if I could change my shape I could regain control over my self-esteem. If I felt more confident about my body I might feel happier about other aspects of my life too.

I asked my doctor about a breast reduction operation. I needed to deal with them because they were a permanent reminder of a bad memory. I told her they were larger than they should be, larger than my waistline, were giving me a bad back and were damaging my posture, making me round my shoulders all the time. I didn't want to tell her that the reason I really wanted it done was because of Linda's cruel taunts.

She told me I was young and my body was still growing. I wouldn't be properly developed until I reached 21. To be fair to her she tried to put me off. Go to the gym, she said. I was already going five days a week, plus I was swimming regularly and dancing at college. There was nothing they could say that would help me improve my general health or physique.

Although she tried to put me off I was persistent, so she referred me to a specialist. He told me if I went ahead at 17 I would be the youngest person in the UK to have it done.

After four appointments I was even more determined. I wanted them gone. Once I was in the system the process was actually quite straightforward. No one challenged me that hard on the psychological reasons why or the impact that having such an operation at that age could mean. Perhaps someone should have referred me for a psychological assessment, which might have revealed the real reasons for me taking such a drastic step. If that had happened maybe I wouldn't have made that decision.

In January 2006, five months before my eighteenth birthday, I was scheduled to have the operation. My breasts were reduced significantly. To give them shape, the surgeon had recommended half-moon implants and as I've grown they will have to be corrected at some point, as is the case with most implants.

I was delighted with the results. It made me feel like a new woman. Physically I no longer identified with the girl Linda had made the subject of her relentless jibes. And, mentally, there was another reason why I felt able to face life's challenges.

Just two weeks before my operation I had some unexpected news. It was Yvonne who broke it to me, after social services had notified her.

Linda was dead.

Persistently plagued with hernia problems, she had

gone in for a routine operation in December 2005. There were complications during the procedure and she died on the operating table.

When Yvonne said the words, 'Linda has passed away,' I just sat there, numb. It was almost too surreal to take in. It had been two years since I'd left the house. Other than that one time I went to her house for lunch, I'd had no direct contact with her. She haunted my dreams, had invaded my psyche and I was due to have an operation to 'correct' slurs she'd made that I could never shake off. To think that now it was over was almost too much for me to get my head around.

'Do you want to go to the funeral?' she asked. It was going to be held in two days' time.

'Yes,' I said immediately. I did, if only to see for myself that she was actually dead.

I had only recently been in touch with Arlene for the first time since leaving the house, so I spoke to her and found out that she and Sara would be going too. Arlene had been living with a boyfriend and was a mother herself now to a little boy and moving on with her life.

Claire had left that social services department so they had assigned me a new social worker called Dawn. She accompanied me to the funeral. I took flowers to give to Linda's family. Despite everything that had gone on, I had always remained fond of them, particularly Terry, her daughter Rebecca and daughter-in-law Deborah. They had been oblivious to Linda's worst behaviour and always tried to be sympathetic to all the girls in her care. I knew they would all be there. It would be a very distressing time for them – to lose their mum, wife and mother-in-law so suddenly and in such tragic circumstances. I wouldn't wish that grief on anyone.

'Stop at mine,' Arlene said, so we made plans to spend some time together after the funeral.

Despite their sorrow, Linda's family were pleased to see me. I imagined they had been kept in the dark about the reasons why the girls and I left. Megan was with them and it was nice to see her again. She had remained in the house all that time, but by all accounts life for her hadn't been quite as bad once we departed.

We were all excited to see each other. We each had our own lives now. Sara was at college, Arlene adjusting to motherhood. Seeing each other again was very emotional. We'd each succeeded in our own small way, after years of being made to feel like nothing. I got a lot of pleasure from seeing Arlene and Sara again. It was strange, though. We had a brief chat about what went on in the house but not a word about how it really affected us. The conversation was restricted to things like, 'Remember the time she did this?' and, 'Can you believe she did that, she was so weird.'

The service was nice. You wouldn't think they were talking about the same person. It was all about how warm she was, how kind-hearted, giving up her home to needy children. If only they knew, I thought. How strange it is that someone can portray such an image and yet the reality is so different.

When the service was over, I paid my respects to her family and was glad to slip away with Arlene, safe in the knowledge that our tormentor really was dead. The circumstances in which she died were tragic. It is a shame that she didn't live to see the error of her ways and at least attempt to undo some of the hurt she caused. But, as I prepared for the next chapter of my life, at least I knew no other child would fall victim to her unfathomable cruelty. No one else need suffer in the Bad Room.

Epilogue

It was April 2014 and I happened to be reading a newspaper. One article caught my eye. It was the story of a woman who had successfully managed to sue a local authority for failing to protect her from her violent, neglectful mother. A landmark case, the paper called it, the first of its kind. Her name was Collette Elliott and she had written a book about her experience. Her story was shocking. She'd suffered years of physical and mental abuse. Social services had been involved from the start. They seemed to know everything that went on, yet they left her with her mother. Years later Collette had managed to get her social work files. They had documented all the meetings held about her welfare and confirmed the many times when she could have been taken out of that destructive situation but wasn't.

Reading her account, I felt compassion for her. It was horrible to think something like that could go on in our civilised society. But my blood also ran cold. I could have been reading about myself. The aspect that jumped out at me were the files. I didn't realise social services kept records on every child in their care. What's more, there was a way to get them. What would mine say? What secrets would they reveal?

I got in touch with Collette, congratulated her on her inspiring story and explained my situation. She couldn't have been more helpful, telling me how she went about it and how best to get hold of my files.

It took a long time and a lot of patience but finally I took delivery of hundreds of pages of A4 paper. The file was filled with copies of documents spanning all the years I was known to social services in two councils. I could scarcely believe what I was seeing. There were entries relating to my mum and dad, to Paul and to Linda.

I had to steel myself before I read them in detail. Did I want to dredge up all the misery I'd spent years trying to forget?

In the years since Linda died I had been through so much. Her death was a watershed moment. The end of a painful chapter. But that wasn't the end of my problems. After leaving college I had a long period of unhappiness. I made a lot of wrong choices and struggled as I tried to find my identity. I battled with my sexuality, tried desperately to decide where I belonged in the world, what my purpose was. Linda had made me want to change the skin I was born in. There were times when I hated myself. I went from being locked in a bedroom and having no freedom, to being allowed to be 'normal'. That was overwhelming. I pushed boundaries, got into relationships that were detrimental and toxic. I didn't know how to be loved and didn't know what love I deserved until my late twenties, and even then I honestly feared I would never see thirty because my mother had lost everything in her life by that age. I had this haunting feeling that I would lose it all too. Only when I chose to get help and began to work on my self-esteem did I begin to see my own worth and work out what my purpose in life was.

Despite these ongoing issues, I managed to forge a career as a business development manager, delivering staff training in the HMP Prison and Education sector. I rekindled my love of dance and fitness, and qualified as a fitness instructor and dance tutor.

I finally got a passport and went travelling for the first time, falling in love with Spain, where I was lucky enough to spend a lot of time.

I managed to become reacquainted with my father, too. On my eighteenth birthday he made attempts through social services to have contact with me again. I was overjoyed to meet him after all those years apart. I'd missed him terribly, but hearing how our enforced separation had taken place was heartbreaking.

Originally my contact with my dad was restricted because my mum controlled the situation. It was a case of if he gave her money he could see me. If not, she would be very volatile towards him. Then the relationship became very strained, even when it came down to foster care.

Before I went into care permanently there was a chance I could have gone to my dad but my mum had stopped that. She still had rights then and she told social services she didn't want my dad having custody of me.

Then when I was in foster care the visits with him stopped because Linda told him I didn't want to see him. She told social services my contact sessions were making me upset. Social services stopped the visits without consulting me to establish if this was the case. When I was made the subject of a section 34:4 order, all contact was stopped.

Only when I turned eighteen was he able to resume contact. He explained that when he was told I didn't want to see him it was upsetting. He didn't like to see me in care and wanted to help but wasn't able to. Hearing all of this was distressing. It was like Linda's final betrayal. Even though she had passed on she still had the capacity to hurt me.

At least he was back in my life, though, and for that I was truly grateful. The relationship with my dad was just one example of the consequences, some unintended, caused by the actions of Linda and social services.

When contact stopped with my mum and dad, so too did the visits with my relatives on each side of the family – and that tarnished those relationships in a way. After becoming reconnected with my dad I saw my grandma again but I just didn't feel like I knew that side of the family anymore. It was more down to me that I didn't pursue any relationship with them. Even though I kept hold of the memories I had, and I knew they were good people, it just seemed that everything that had happened over the years made me put up barriers and I couldn't force myself to be close to them again. My sense was that I'd managed so long without them, so even when my grandma passed I didn't feel I could go to the funeral. I supported my dad but I said, 'I hope you can understand, I just feel like an outcast.' Other family members asked me if I was going and my dad sent me photos of her house, which showed she always kept photos of me on display, which broke my heart, I just felt so disconnected from that side of the family – apart from my dad.

The same went for my mother's side. I only reconnected with my grandma once I'd moved in with Yvonne. I went to see her once or twice and we started building up a relationship because I could go out at weekends and see my family, something I was never allowed to do with Linda.

But when I was going through my emotional turmoil I stopped contact. The last I heard from her was a voicemail asking me to call her back. I didn't respond and a few weeks later my social worker called to tell me she had passed away. I was devastated I hadn't been emotionally closer, as I would have called. I'll never know if she knew she was ill and wanted to speak to me, aware that it might be the last time.

I did go to her funeral and was excited to be able to see my Auntie Marie, who I hadn't seen or heard from in so many years. When I arrived I asked some relatives, 'Where's Marie?' There was a horrible moment when they exchanged glances, shocked expressions on their faces. 'Marie's died as well,' one said.

She had passed away only a few months before from liver disease. She was only 27. Grandma was going to be buried with her. I was doubly devastated, as Marie had been one of the rare shining lights of happiness amid the darkness. I couldn't believe I would never see her again.

And so, by the time I sat down and prepared to read my files I was plagued by mixed emotions, but overriding everything was a desire to see for myself what had really happened – and why.

As if looking through the pages, reading about your own life, wasn't hard enough, the job hadn't been made easy for me. The files were not in chronological order; some sections were redacted, and within them there were also pictures of another girl called Jade. They'd clearly mixed up the files. Was that going to be an indication of the muddled thinking throughout the social services departments that dealt with my situation?

Reading my reports I learned that social services became involved with my wellbeing from the age of three, when Paul came into Mum's life. Right from the early days there were concerns that I had witnessed domestic violence between them. This I must have blacked out as I could only remember their blazing rows, not the resulting physical violence.

Social workers requested my mother break up with Paul but she wouldn't. I was regularly tested and found to be malnourished and underweight. Social workers had to take me to a children's hospital. Clearly Mum wasn't coping. I knew her personality changed dramatically when Paul was around and when he went away, but now I read that she was bi-polar and suffered from other mental illnesses. That explained some of her behaviour but I couldn't help having feelings of bitterness when I read about some of the incidents I had blacked out for years because they were so painful.

There was the day when Paul held me hostage with Mum, the police and social services outside the house. It was documented how he smashed the house up and rammed my face into a picture frame and how Mum took me to hospital where I received treatment for facial injuries. Looking in the mirror I realised that the marks on my face that I still have today were a permanent reminder of that terrible day. Reading about it brought flooding back the memories I had suppressed, and I wept for the poor child that had to live through that.

What I didn't understand was why social services didn't remove me from my mother at this point when surely they had recognised my home life was unsafe? Recorded also were the times Paul was violent to my mother and social services moved us into women's refuges, but she always went back to him. Mum clearly manipulated the situation so she could keep her children. She routinely failed to comply with their requests yet kept getting another chance. When my brother and sister were a little older the reports multiplied. There was documented information on physical and mental abuse, neglect, being malnourished. I do not understand why social services did not remove us from her care. I was interested to read there were times – earlier than I could remember – when I was placed with foster carers on a temporary basis, but this was more as respite for my mother and we were always returned to her.

Social workers recognised that I had had to grow up fast, that mum treated me like an adult and I had to effectively look after Jack and Ellen, taking on responsibilities no child that age should have been expected to do.

It was distressing to read that so many instances of abuse and neglect were documented without any real action being taken. Mum used to ring them and say,

'Oh, I've hit Jade again,' and they would come round, document that, take the reports, speak to me, take me to hospital if needed, and yet I'd be left to stay with my mum. On several occasions that happened and none of it was considered serious enough for them to say, 'Actually, she can't stay with you.'

It made me wonder what would have had to happen to me for them to take action?

It's not like the problems were hidden; Mum hadn't been the only person who had reported what had been going on. My grandma rang them on several occasions to tell them her daughter had hit me. The council joiner reported that he came to the house and found Mum had locked Jack in the bedroom. The door was held shut and he was trying to get out. Neighbours reported their concerns. At various times, one or all three of us siblings were seen running about outside with no shoes on, sometimes very late at night. There was an occasion I recalled when I had approached the car I knew belonged to a social worker and asked her if she could put me in foster care, but she drove off.

Social workers had documented all of this information, that had been passed to them in black and white, so what was going on? Were there line managers who were too scared to make a decision?

As the years went on, social services knew that Mum had become a heroin user. One of the most distressing events for me to read about was the day when our house was raided by police. Mum had breached bail conditions. This was another occasion I had partially blocked out of my mind. There were times when I questioned my own memory. Had Mum really asked me to take a pencil case filled with drugs and needles? It almost seemed too reckless to be true. Yet, there it was, written down in front of me. The operation even had a name. Reading the social worker's report into the incident only reinforced my disgust at my mother trying to get me to put the stationery case into my bag, I think in her head she thought I would have known to dispose of it. Sad as it is to admit, I probably would have done.

My paperwork showed every photocopy of food grants given to my mother so she could feed her children, yet still I had had to go to the doctor's surgery to get free hot chocolate. Our education suffered because of my mother. We constantly changed schools and in one year we hadn't attended class at all. At one point a remark was made by a social worker, as she asked when was the last time I went to school.

What my files showed was that everyone was talking about our situation but no one did anything. You can't have an adult smash a child's face into a picture frame and put that child back into that same environment.

It seemed like a great weight was put on my reluctance to speak, but I knew not to speak to anyone because I knew it would get my mum into trouble. I was also always questioned by my mum on what had happened, what they'd asked. She schooled me not to tell them that Paul was there. I felt loyalty to my mum and I didn't want to get her into trouble.

When I looked back it had been such a stressful time. I didn't ever feel like a normal child. I'd look at everyone else playing in the playground, who seemed not to have a care in the world. I had this thing where I had to protect my mum, everyone was questioning me and I was defensive all the time. I was guarded and I was probably an angry little child. I was always aware that I couldn't relax and just be a child. There was embarrassment as well. I was always taken out of class and being questioned. I never had a normal relationship with a teacher. It was like everyone interrogated me. They all wanted to know something.

It was like that from day one. There was never a golden period. In my head I always used to think my mum changed when drugs came into our lives, but the reality was her behaviour was an issue long before that.

Initially, I had come under the care of one social services department and this transferred to another neighbouring authority when I went into foster care. At first they sent me to Linda only on a temporary basis. Discussions were held about whether all three of us should be kept together but they decided to keep me separate because I needed some respite as I had taken on the mother role, feeding and clothing my siblings.

This course of action would dictate our future foster care arrangements as it was always considered best that Jack and Ellen stay together and I go somewhere else on my own. This ultimately led to me being the subject of a different care order.

When I went to Linda it was as I had remembered it. I was happy to be there at the start because she offered a welcome change from the chaotic life I'd known up until then. The incident that my mother reported was documented but the outcome seemed very much that it was put on me to decide. How can a ten-year-old girl know best? I had confirmed she'd hit me. Linda even admitted it herself. Why was there not a stronger course of action? They just seemed keen to sweep it under the carpet and once Linda established her strict routine we were done for.

It was emotionally exhausting, reading all the harrowing details of my life. My whole childhood was documented from 1994. I was abused, neglected and listed as a high-risk case who was likely to receive physical harm from my own parents. I just kept thinking why did it take social services so long to actually intervene? And when they eventually did remove me from my parents they still allowed me to be abused by my foster mother.

Once I'd read all the documents I was in no doubt that they revealed from start to finish where social services had gone wrong and how I was failed by them.

I didn't have nor was I allowed to have a normal upbringing, and after a failed suicide attempt and years of depression I was surprised I'd actually managed to make something of my life. I realised I'd got to where I was through the love and support of friends and an inner belief I had in myself. Somehow, despite everything, I'd had the determination not to become another hopeless failed statistic. I didn't want to let other people's failings be the reason why I didn't succeed.

When I thought of Linda and how she behaved I just kept thinking: how had this woman ever become a foster carer? If the information about her own damaged childhood was true then shouldn't she have been psychologically assessed to establish she was fit to look after children? Just because someone wants to take in children doesn't mean they should.

One of the most distressing aspects of my files concerned Arlene and Sara. There was mention of things they'd suffered when they were very young. When I read that I called Sara, explained how I had found out and asked her if it was true. She confirmed that it was true. It was extremely upsetting to think they had gone through years of that and then Linda used the very reason they had been placed in foster care against them. I thought of all the times she had called Arlene and Sara horrible names, saying nasty things about them. It was absolutely heartbreaking.

I came away from reading the files with an over-whelming sense that someone should be held account-able for failing to protect me. I found a law firm willing to take on the case and after they spent a few months looking over the documents they came back with the news that they felt there was potential for two claims, against both councils.

The claim against the first council, whose actions led me to be fostered by Linda, alleged that had they discharged their duty of care my siblings and I would have been removed in the mid-1990s and I would have avoided three further years of neglect and emotional and physical abuse.

The claim against the other alleged similar failings.

Regarding Linda, there had never been another discussion about pressing charges since the initial one social services had with me. Apart from Arlene, Sara and me being removed from her care, she suffered no punishment.

When I was putting together my claims I got in touch with Arlene and Sara to tell them what I was doing. The same lawyers put in claims for them too, against the second council. In September 2018 we were all offered settlements from that council and in May 2020 the first council also agreed to settle my claim. The settlements did not come with admissions of responsibility but it was an amazing feeling to be vindi-cated. It had been an ordeal to read through my paperwork but it was worth it. The settlements in no way compensated for all the abuse I had suffered but at least it showed I had been right to raise the actions.

Arlene and Sara received payouts too. Tragically for Arlene she never got a chance to enjoy it. She had gone on to become a mother to two young children, but not long before the settlement was reached she was found to have breast cancer. Doctors operated on her but it later returned and this time spread to other parts of her body. She was only 32 when she died. Her story is one of heartbreak and hardship. From what she suffered in her early life, to having to endure daily torment at Linda's to then battling cancer, knowing she was going to leave two young children motherless, it must have felt like one long struggle for her. At least before she died she knew she'd received money that would help the children she loved. That was something.

According to Local Government Association figures, in the past decade the number of children in care in England has risen 28 per cent to a ten-year high. As the numbers rise the chances for good outcomes for children in care continue to drop. Some children aren't strong enough to cope with their situations and often turn to alcohol and drugs as they become teenagers, not getting any real help to deal with their problems. There has also been a reduction in the amount of money that local government has received over that ten-year period to assign to children's services, despite the fact that societal pressures are leading to more family breakdowns.

What concerns me is that the highest increase in need is in the age group of children ten years old and upwards – the age at which I became the subject of a care order.

It is not all doom and gloom, though. There are lots of good people working in the care system. Shona and Claire, who were my social workers for years, were kind to me. When I was finally removed from Linda's house, Claire was very happy. In my reports I saw that she had said it was not a safe environment, but whoever was higher up in the chain was not acting on her assessment. Arlene and Sara told me a similar story. Their social worker was saying the same sort of thing but those making the decisions didn't seem to agree.

I'm sure within social services departments up and down the country the people on the frontline are trying to make a difference. It is up to the powers that be to give them their support – and hopefully that will happen by reading accounts from people like me, people who have been through the system and who have found the courage and means to have their voices heard.

A start is being made. The government has pledged to review children's care. It is boosting the number of foster and adoptive parents and is setting aside £45 million in a new fund to improve outcomes. After reports showed that children who have access to extended families do better than those cut off from their relatives, more is being done to develop kinships. Without that the reality is that too many children feel isolated and stigmatised.

I know this only too well. My relationship with the brother and sister I adore was severely affected by our enforced separation. When I was at Linda's our contact dried up for months. Lack of social workers or Linda claiming she was too ill meant contact meetings were cancelled at short notice. It was only when I moved to Yvonne's that regular contact was resumed.

By then it was strange to see how much they'd grown. Jack was 6ft 2in and towered over all of us. My sister, although then a teenager, still liked to be glued to my hip. Since we reconnected we hung out at Jack's house, watched movies and tried to make up for all that lost time.

They don't know all that I went through. There were some things I wanted to protect them from, but they now respect my need to write about my experience.

I have not had any contact with Paul Harries. From my files I saw that he was in and out of prison throughout my childhood and the last I heard he was in very poor health.

As for my mum, I have had intermittent contact with her over the years, the last being around three years ago. My views on her are complicated. When I thought about the letters from her to me while I was at Linda's, asking me to 'remember the good', I felt she was still trying to manipulate my feelings.

But having worked with people with mental health issues and knowing now that my mum has been diagnosed with schizophrenia I can see that she had been battling problems for years. I have some sympathy for her now because perhaps the help she needed back then simply wasn't there. There wasn't the same education or understanding around mental health issues that there is today, either. She didn't know how to deal with her problems, so they were passed on to her children.

Hers is a tragic story. She lost five children; three of us were taken into care and two others were put up for adoption. She wasn't equipped to be a mother and couldn't cope with the responsibilities it brought. It must have been overwhelming for her.

As for me, for years I thought of myself as quite a strong person and was probably guilty of being blasé about what went on because I felt I just had to get over it. But it's only now, as I've started talking and writing about what happened, that I realise so much went on that needs to be aired.

In some ways the legacy of my experience in foster care lives on. I still struggle with my self-image due to what I went through, but it's something I am aware of and have found a way to manage it.

On the whole, though, I have tried to be positive and take that mindset into everything I do. In 2015, while watching a television programme on surrogacy and IVF, an account from a woman whose only chance of having a family was down to the generosity of an egg donor gripped me. Here was a woman choosing a difficult path because she wanted to love and nurture a child of her own. It was a dream for her. So moved was I by her story that I decided I wanted to be able to help a family like hers. I contacted Care Fertility and started the process. I went through counselling, various tests and a thorough screening process to ensure this was the right thing for me to do. Once selected, I started hormone treatment and over three years donated eggs five times. Care Fertility only notify donors when there has been a successful live birth but I am delighted to say that since then they have notified me on four occasions, each time sending flowers as a thank you. It is always an overwhelming feeling knowing I've helped give a family a special gift. I used to feel ashamed of my life. I never told anyone anything about my past. It was a closed book. It is vitally important that people who have gone through the care system and had a bad experience speak out. Collette's story helped me and I hope that if my story helps one other person to think and talk about their experiences then I have achieved my goal.

I fought for years to make something of my life and not become another lost cause in the social service system. I want this story to come from a place of strength. I want anyone who reads my book and has experienced the same failings in the system to realise that not everyone is a victim. Everyone has a choice – to let their past define them or their future, or not. I hope my story helps people find the strength to fight for what they want in life.

Acknowledgements

First of all, I would like to thank Doug for hearing my story and helping me share it with the world. Without you this would not have been possible and for that I will be eternally grateful. Thank you to my agent Andrew Lownie and HarperCollins for giving me an amazing platform to share my life with an audience, in the hope that it will change one person's life and give them the strength to tell their story.

Thank you to Collette Elliott – because of your story I found the strength to fight for justice and tell mine.

To my brother and sister, J and R. There is not a day that goes by when I do not think of you, and I can't tell you how proud I am of you both. I love you both dearly – never forget that. 'From chaos came perfection.'

Thank you to my friends D, N, V, V, K, R and R. You girls were my happy place, filled with laughter and mischievous memories. You were my escape and the reason I am sitting here writing this today. You saved me without knowing it.

Daniel and Jayne, thank you for living through my teenage years with me and bringing me into your family, sharing laughter and love. You allowed me to find and be myself without ever judging me. Daniel, thank you for always making me feel like the only girl on the dance floor. Both of you will always have the largest place in my heart.

Kayleigh Holden – thank you for all your loyalty, laughter and memories. I hope I get to live my remaining years having you as my best friend. Thank you for always being on my side no matter what.

Patricia, Chris and Karen – I was brought into your family and you instantly smothered me with love and kindness. You showed me how to accept love – a love with no ulterior motive. You made me believe I could always achieve what I wanted in life with hard work, and with that I never stopped working.

Melanie Bullock, thank you to my best friend. Thank you for always being on the other end of the phone for four-hour talks. Thank you for always being there through dark times and happy times. Thank you for giving me the best thirtieth birthday a girl could ask for. For a girl who never thought she would live past her thirties, you gave me the happiest day I could ever have imagined – I love you.

Rachel and Sally – the love I have for you both is unfathomable. Thank you from the bottom of my heart for all your support over the years. You are not only my friends – you are my family and I love you both.

Sally Robinson – thank you for always making me laugh until it hurts, for being the person I can look at and instantly we both know what the other is thinking. Thank you for being as wonderfully weird as me. Forever my FWEND.

Lauren C (Fave) – thank you for the years of friendship. No matter what we have been through, we have supported each other or egged each other on. We have grown together and found strength in each other. Thank you for midnight talks on the Universe and the Law of Attraction – Moons & Moons, Stars & Stars.

Chloe, my soulmate, my partner in crime – thank you for coming into my life and showing me an unconditional love, guiding me, supporting me and helping me to believe anything is possible, should I want it enough. Thank you for filling the hardest of days with pure love – 'I could get used to this.'

Thank you to my sisters J and D. This story is for you both. It's our story. We shared the hardest of times together. We went through things that no child should ever go through. I believe that our love and our sisterhood got us through it all. D, you were taken before your time. I hope you're up in heaven singing and dancing and your soul is at peace – until we meet again, Sister.

To my Dad (Moon Head) – I love you – forever your daughter.

To my readers, the silent voices and inside warriors, to anyone who has endured the same failings in the system. I hope you find strength in my story to find your voice and tell yours. I hope you read my story and you are inspired. I hope that you dig down inside yourself and realise your potential and worth. Find your passion in life and you will find your purpose. Turn your trauma into your strength. How we respond in life will determine what life we live. Give love and accept love.